WHAT YOU I

————— AE

CANCER, CHEMO AND COPING

CHEMO
CONUERSATIONS

Advice from a Cancer Doctor

Angela DeRidder, MD, MPH

Chemo Conversations: What You Need to Know About Cancer, Chemo and Coping—Advice from a Cancer Doctor

Published by Chemo Conversations, LLC
Salisbury, MD
www.chemoconversations.com

Library of Congress Control Number 2021900475

ISBN (paperback) 978-1-7362529-0-1
ISBN (ebook) 978-1-7362529-1-8

Cover design by Klassic Designs
Interior design by Josep Book Designs

To my husband, Stephen, and my daughter, Grace.
I love you.

To my patients.
Thank you for letting me be part of your lives.

Table of Contents

Introduction

Ms. Elizabeth sat in my office, twisting her hands nervously.

"Hello," I said, walking into the room. "My name is Dr. DeRidder. Do you know why your primary care doctor sent you here today?" I took a seat at the computer. Across from me, the middle-aged woman sat rigidly in her chair, holding her husband's hand. She appeared to be in excellent health.

Ms. Elizabeth blinked rapidly, trying to clear away tears. "Yes. My doctor said I might have..." she swallowed hard. "He said I have cancer." Her face crumpled and her husband quickly squeezed her hand.

I reached over to take her free hand. "Okay," I said. "Let's start at the beginning."

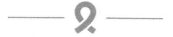

Every day, I see patients just like Ms. Elizabeth in my office; scared and overwhelmed, they walk into my office uncertain of what the future might bring. Cancer is a life-changing, shocking, terrible thing. It changes plans, dreams, and lives. As a chemotherapy doctor, also known as a medical oncologist, one of the most common emotions I encounter in patients is *fear*—fear of chemotherapy, fear of side effects, and fear of the future. Much of this fear stems from the unknown. Learning that you have cancer is like being dropped off in the wilderness without a map. Without understanding the path ahead, it is easy to feel overwhelmed and out of control.

This is why I wrote this book.

I wrote it in hopes that I can alleviate some of your fears, to guide you through the wilderness. As a practicing medical oncologist, I interact with cancer patients every day. Through countless conversations with my patients, I have determined one very important, life-altering fact: Knowledge is power. Knowledge is *choice*. By understanding your diagnosis and treatment options, you will be better prepared to make decisions about your cancer care.

Unfortunately, sometimes these important cancer conversations do not happen. In my practice, the biggest constraint to these conversations is *time*. In today's health care culture, most doctor visits are arranged in 15 to 20 minute time intervals. As anyone who has ever had a doctor's visit can attest, 15 minutes is simply not enough time to discuss all the topics needed to maintain your health, let alone begin to navigate the complex and difficult topic of cancer.

By writing this book, I hope to provide you, and hopefully all cancer patients, some much-needed information about cancer, chemotherapy, and your changing health. This book contains much of the knowledge you need to make informed decisions about your future. In addition, it contains all the tips and tricks I have learned over my career that will help you manage your chemotherapy side effects with confidence. My hope is that this book will serve as your trail markers, rations, and a guiding light while finding your way through the wilderness of a cancer diagnosis.

WHAT YOU WILL GET OUT OF THIS BOOK

In this book, I will cover the basics about cancer treatment. I will discuss the rationale behind surgery, chemotherapy, and radiation, and why we use these treatments. I will cover the potential side effects of chemotherapy, as well as how to manage these side effects. Finally, I will discuss how to navigate living with the physical, emotional, and financial implications of cancer. Throughout these discussions, I will highlight the stories of real patients I have treated and walked with on this difficult and emotional journey.[1]

It is important to emphasize that while I am a cancer doctor, I am not a cancer survivor. All the issues discussed in this book will be from a cancer doctor's perspective. It is true that I have not walked in your shoes. However, I have walked beside hundreds of patients on a journey similar to yours. The topics covered in this book are topics I discuss with my patients every single day.

---

[1] Patient ages and names have been changed to maintain privacy.

Chapter 1: Starting at the beginning	The basic concepts behind cancer staging, chemotherapy/ immunotherapy, surgery and radiation, and how these therapies are used to treat cancer.
Chapter 2: Making the most out of your consult appointment	How to prepare for your appointment, whom to bring, and whom to tell about your cancer diagnosis.
Chapter 3: Chemotherapy side effects	The most common side effects of chemotherapy and methods to anticipate and alleviate them.
Chapter 4: Understanding your labs	Which labs your oncologist will monitor during treatment and how to improve them.
Chapter 5: Life during cancer treatment	How to improve the relationship between you and your doctor, as well as maintain your emotional, physical, and financial health.
Chapter 6: Survivorship	A brief introduction to the concept of survivorship.
Chapter 7: Stage 4 cancer	Special information for patients diagnosed with stage 4 cancer.

Please keep in mind that while this book will cover the basics about cancer and cancer treatment, there are many topics regarding cancer care that I will not cover. I chose to limit the information in this book to make it compact, digestible, and relatable. The goal of this book is not to replace your meetings with your cancer care team, but to supplement your appointments with additional information. If you have questions about your cancer care that are not addressed in this book, please discuss them with your oncologist. If you have questions about topics that *are* addressed in this book, also discuss them with your oncologist! Remember while I am a cancer doctor, I am not *your* cancer doctor. All information provided in this book is intended for educational purposes and not intended to diagnose or treat any condition. While the information in this book is general and can be applied to most patients, everyone is different, and any changes to your medications, diet, and exercise regimen should be cleared with your oncologist first.

Now, as I told Ms. Elizabeth, let's start at the beginning.

First, we must understand what we are facing.

CHAPTER 1

Starting at the Beginning

"All right," I told Ms. Elizabeth. "I've reviewed the records your surgeon sent over, so I have a good understanding of what's happened over the past couple of months. I'm going to review what my understanding is and fill me in if there is anything that I missed.

"It looks like a month ago you noticed a lump in your left breast. You went to your primary care doctor, and they ordered a mammogram. That mammogram came back showing an abnormality in the left breast, so they referred you to a breast surgeon. Your breast surgeon did a biopsy, and that's what came back confirming breast cancer in the left breast."

Ms. Elizabeth nodded in agreement.

"Your surgeon did a partial resection of your breast, and that came back confirming breast cancer, and it was what we call 'estrogen receptor positive, progesterone receptor positive, and HER-2 negative.' Does that sound familiar?" I asked.

"Yes," replied Ms. Elizabeth, "But I don't really understand what that means. Can you explain that?"

"Sure," I said. "All breast tissue relies on female hormones, estrogen and progesterone. That's how your breast tissue knows when you hit puberty, it's how your breast tissue knows to make milk during pregnancy. All breast tissue has receptors for these female hormones. However, about 80% of breast cancers actually express an overabundance of receptors. These breast cancers will actually bind to your female hormones and use them as a food source, almost like a fuel. Does that make sense so far?"

Ms. Elizabeth and her husband looked at each other and nodded.

"We test all breast cancers for these receptors, and yours came back positive, telling us that your cancer is feeding off your female hormones of estrogen and progesterone. This is important because it influences how we treat your cancer."

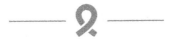

I consider our first appointment together extremely important. Much like I did with Ms. Elizabeth, during your initial appointment, I will sit down with you and share vital information about your cancer. Typically, I will discuss the type of cancer you have, the stage, treatment options, side effects, and the expected outcome.

My initial consult appointment generally follows the below format:

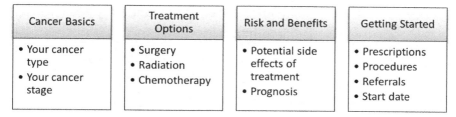

Figure 1. My typical initial consult format.

Every doctor will approach a consult appointment differently, and of course, there is no right or wrong approach. However, regardless of the flow of your doctor's visit, I believe that each of the above topics should be touched on at some point during your conversation. If your doctor does not bring up one of these topics, I would encourage you to inquire about whatever information you need. Your oncologist is here to help you. If you have questions, he or she will be happy to provide more details.

The purpose of this chapter is to explain some of the basics your cancer doctor will be discussing during your initial appointment. I will discuss **cancer staging** and the rationale behind **surgery, chemotherapy/immunotherapy,** and **radiation**. I'll cover an extremely important concept known as **"performance status."** Finally, I will discuss how your cancer stage and your performance status all weigh into determining your overall **prognosis.**

WHAT YOU WILL GET OUT OF THIS CHAPTER

Cancer staging	How your cancer doctor determines your cancer stage, and why it is important.
Treatment options	The rationale behind surgery, radiation and chemotherapy/ immunotherapy.
Performance status	Understanding the concept of performance status.
Prognosis	How your doctor determines your prognosis.

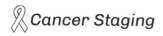 Cancer Staging

Cancer staging may seem complicated, and it can be. However, while the intricacies of cancer staging may differ depending on the type of cancer, there are typically four stages of cancer.

Cancer Staging Made Simple		
Stage	**Explanation**	**Example**
Stage 1	Cancer is small and still within the organ it first started.	A small colon cancer. No lymph nodes involved.
Stage 2	Cancer is larger but still within the organ it first started. Alternatively, cancer is small but there are cancer cells found in nearby lymph nodes.	A large colon cancer. No lymph nodes involved.
Stage 3	Cancer is very large or cancer cells are found in distant lymph nodes	A colon cancer with evidence of cancer in lymph nodes within the abdomen.
Stage 4	Cancer has traveled from the organ in which it first started to another organ.	Colon cancer that has spread to the liver.

Please note that the explanation above is very general, and there are many exceptions to this explanation. Every cancer is staged slightly differently, and staging can depend on factors not included in this table. For these reasons, it is extremely important to discuss the stage of your cancer with your oncologist.

Why is staging so important? Cancer staging affects the way we approach cancer treatment. Typically, the smaller and more localized a cancer, the more likely your doctor is to recommend surgery. The goal with surgery is to cut the cancer out and leave no cancer behind. If your cancer is small, it is easy for your surgeon to accomplish that goal. The more the cancer spreads out, the more likely your doctors are to recommend additional or alternative therapies, such as radiation and chemotherapy.

Cancer staging also affects prognosis. All treatments for early stage cancer, from surgery to radiation to chemotherapy, are designed to prevent cancer cells from entering the blood system. Once cancer enters the blood system, it can use the blood system like a highway to travel to other organs. If you have a large cancer or cancer involving your lymph nodes, your risk for cancer entering the blood system is higher. The higher the chance that cancer has entered the blood system, typically the higher the cancer stage, and the poorer the prognosis.

Your oncologist should tell you your cancer stage. If your oncologist does not discuss your cancer stage, please ask. Because of its implications for your treatment as well as prognosis, it is important for you to understand the stage of your cancer. Initially, the stage of your cancer may be unknown and may require further scans or biopsies. This is common. Sometimes, you will only know the final stage of your cancer after you have your cancer removed.

Ultimately, however, your cancer doctor should be able to provide you with the stage of your cancer, your treatment plan, and your prognosis.

Treatment Options

As mentioned, your cancer treatment highly depends on your cancer stage. Stages 1, 2, and 3 cancers are considered early stage cancers. If you have early stage cancer, likely your cancer doctor will recommend either surgery or radiation, possibly followed by chemotherapy, all with the goal of reducing the risk of your cancer coming back in the future. If you were diagnosed with stage 4 cancer or **"metastatic"** cancer, the goal of treatment is different. You can learn more about stage 4 cancer treatment in Chapter 7.

Typically with early stage cancer, there are three different treatment approaches—surgery, radiation, and chemotherapy. Below, I will review the role for each approach.

Surgery

The goal of surgery is to remove the bulk of your cancer. The less cancer in your body, the better. Your surgeon, or **surgical oncologist**, will be a physician who specializes in removing cancer using a scalpel in the operating room. If your surgeon thinks that he or she can safely remove your cancer without hurting the surrounding tissues, he or she will remove as much cancer as possible.

However, cancer cells are microscopic. By the time a tumor can be seen on a scan or by the naked eye, that tumor is already made up of thousands of cancer cells. Even if your surgeon removes all visible tumors, even if all your margins were negative, the concern is always that a couple of small, microscopic cancer cells could have been left behind. Unfortunately, cancer is like a weed—if you leave the roots behind, it will grow back again. If there is one cancer cell left behind, eventually, there could be thousands.

That is where radiation and chemotherapy come in.

Radiation

Radiation is a form of cancer treatment that focuses radiation beams on a specific part of the body. The most likely place for cancer to grow back is the place where it first started. With radiation, your **radiation oncologist** will use radiation beams to kill cancer cells in the area where your cancer initially grew. Like surgery, radiation typically touches just one area—the area where the beams are focused. Your radiation doctor cannot give radiation to your entire body, as it would be too toxic. But he or she can use focused radiation beams to treat the area where the cancer first grew, to try to kill any lingering cancer cells.

Both surgery and radiation are "local" therapies, meaning that the treatment affects just one area of the body. What about the rest of the body? What about cancer cells trying to spread to other organs?

As mentioned, cancer spreads through the blood system. A tiny cancer cell will break off from the tumor, and travel through the blood system, using it like a highway. Once cancer enters the blood system, it can go anywhere. To prevent this from happening, you need a treatment that can *also* go anywhere. You need chemotherapy.

Chemotherapy

Chemotherapy is the use of intravenous or oral medications to kill cancer cells. Your **medical oncologist** is a doctor who specializes in safely administering chemotherapy and cancer-killing medications. Chemotherapy is a "systemic" treatment, meaning that the medications enter into the blood system and circulate around your entire body. Because chemotherapy enters into the blood system, anywhere the blood goes, the treatment goes as well. By giving chemotherapy, your medical oncologist can reduce the risk of cancer spreading out into the body and coming back in the future.

One important concept in cancer treatment is the *timing* of chemotherapy. Chemotherapy given after surgery is known as *adjuvant* **chemotherapy**, and chemotherapy given before surgery is known as *neoadjuvant* **chemotherapy**.

Before Surgery: Neoadjuvant Chemotherapy

Chemotherapy administered prior to surgery is called "neoadjuvant chemotherapy." The concept behind neoadjuvant chemotherapy is to shrink the cancer as much as possible before surgery.

As mentioned, the goal with surgery is to remove the cancer and leave no cancer behind. However, sometimes the cancer is growing in a delicate area, making surgery risky. Sometimes the cancer is so large or spread out that removing all the cancer would be harmful to your body. In these situations, we give chemotherapy before surgery in an attempt to shrink the cancer as much as possible. Then your surgeon will go in and remove your cancer.

Imagine a flower garden with a knot of weeds growing in the middle. You could dig up the knot of weeds, but it will leave a large hole in your garden and potentially damage some of the healthy flowers.

So instead, you spray weed killer on your garden. The weed killer kills off some of the weeds growing in your garden, shrinking the clump of weeds to a more manageable size. Now that you have shrunk the clump of weeds to a manageable size, you can dig it up. So you go get your shovel and dig up the clump of weeds. You have now eliminated the weeds from your garden and preserved your flowers. You have used neoadjuvant weed killer.

MS. KATIE'S STORY

Ms. Katie was a 50-year-old woman with two areas of breast cancer in her left breast. One mass measured 7cm at the time of her diagnosis, and the other measured 3cm. She also had a large lymph node palpable under her left arm, which, when biopsied, was positive for breast cancer. One method to treat her cancer would be to remove the entire left breast, as well as the lymph nodes under her left arm. However, Ms. Katie was very concerned about proceeding with surgery. To her, keeping her left breast intact was essential to her femininity and her overall self-esteem. If at all possible, she wished to undergo partial breast removal as opposed to complete removal of the left breast.

Given her large breast tumor, the presence of a positive lymph node, and her desire to preserve her breast, I elected to give her neoadjuvant chemotherapy, or chemotherapy before surgery. The goal was to shrink her cancer as much as possible, allowing her surgeon to remove only as much breast as absolutely necessary. Markers were placed in her breast cancer and the abnormal lymph node so that her surgeon would know exactly where her cancer was originally located.

She tolerated chemotherapy well, and had dramatic shrinkage of her left breast tumor. After she completed chemotherapy, she proceeded with surgery. A review of the surgical specimen showed no active cancer cells. Her breast cancer had completely responded to chemotherapy.

Given that her breast cancer was aggressive and her risk of recurrence was high, after healing from her surgery she was referred for radiation. She underwent radiation to the left breast and lymph nodes with minimal side effects. At this time, she is currently two years out from her initial cancer diagnosis and remains breast cancer free.

Ms. Katie's situation stresses an important concept regarding neoadjuvant chemotherapy. Neoadjuvant chemotherapy can have remarkable results. Cancers may completely disappear on scans and even disappear under the microscope. However, the majority of cancers cannot be cured with chemotherapy alone.[2] Chemotherapy can kill cancer cells—but it cannot *permanently* kill cancer cells. Once the chemotherapy stops, at some point, the cancer will grow back. For that reason, neoadjuvant chemotherapy is always followed by what we call **definitive therapy**—surgery or radiation.

After Surgery: Adjuvant Chemotherapy

Adjuvant chemotherapy is chemotherapy given *after* surgery. As discussed, the goal with surgery is to remove as much cancer as safely possible. However, sometimes surgeons find evidence that cancer is trying to creep into the blood system. Sometimes a cancer is known to be very aggressive, with a high chance of coming back in the future. Whenever surgery and radiation are not enough to reduce the risk of cancer recurring or spreading, adjuvant chemotherapy is typically recommended.

---

[2] Exceptions include leukemia and lymphoma, which can often be cured with chemotherapy alone.

One common scenario requiring adjuvant chemotherapy is cancer involving lymph nodes. Lymph nodes are clusters of immune cells that sit in various areas of your body. Like cop cars sitting at the side of the road watching for speeding cars, lymph nodes sit next to your blood system and monitor your blood for suspicious activity. If a lymph node sees something abnormal in your blood system, it captures it and tries to eliminate it. For example, if you have a sore throat, you may develop swollen lymph nodes in your neck. The lymph nodes in your neck are capturing bacteria that have entered your blood system from your throat. The immune cells in your lymph nodes multiply, kill the bacteria, and then return to normal.

If cancer cells leak into your blood system from a tumor, typically, the nearest lymph nodes will capture the cells. However, while lymph nodes can capture cancer cells, they cannot *kill* cancer cells. So if you have lymph nodes positive for cancer, there is a high chance that some cancer cells are *still* remaining in the blood system. For this reason, adjuvant chemotherapy will likely be recommended.

If your cancer was large, this also raises the risk of cancer cells entering the blood system. This is simply due to sheer volume. The more cancer cells present, the higher the likelihood that a cell can break off and enter the blood system. Finally, if you have an aggressive form of cancer, chemotherapy may be discussed even if your cancer was small, or your lymph nodes were not involved.

In summary, if you have had surgery and your cancer was found to be aggressive or present in your lymph nodes, there is a high likelihood your oncologist will recommend adjuvant chemotherapy. The goal of your adjuvant chemotherapy is to kill cancer cells in the blood system and reduce the risk of your cancer coming back.

MS. STEPHANIE'S STORY

Ms. Stephanie was a 44-year-old woman with stage 2 left-sided breast cancer. She underwent removal of her left breast, as well as removal of lymph nodes under her left arm. Three out of ten lymph nodes from under her left arm were found to be positive for breast cancer. Based on this, her breast surgeon referred her to my office to discuss adjuvant chemotherapy.

"I don't understand," she said with frustration. "My surgeon said that he got all the cancer."

I explained to her that, yes, her surgeon had removed the cancer completely. All her margins were negative. However, the presence of cancer in her lymph nodes told me that at some point, cancer cells had tried to escape into her blood system. Though her surgeon had removed her breast tumor as well as the cancerous lymph nodes, there was a small chance that cancer cells could be floating in her blood system, trying to cause trouble for the future.

"Without chemotherapy," I told her, "There is 30 percent chance that your cancer will come back in the next 10 years. With chemotherapy, that chance decreases to 15 percent."

After hearing the numbers and discussing potential side effects, Ms. Stephanie decided to move forward with adjuvant chemotherapy. She has since completed her chemotherapy as well as radiation to the left breast and lymph nodes, and is currently living cancer free.

Immunotherapy

An important type of systemic therapy that bears mentioning is something known as immunotherapy. Immunotherapy is also considered a form of "systemic" therapy. Much like chemotherapy, immunotherapy is a medicine that can be administered before or after surgery to affect cancer cells. However, immunotherapy works very differently than chemotherapy, and these differences are worth highlighting.

As mentioned, chemotherapy is a chemical that kills cells— often indiscriminately. Most chemotherapy agents cannot distinguish between a cancer cell or a normal, healthy cell in your body. Many of the side effects that can occur from chemotherapy, such as hair loss, mouth sores, and diarrhea, happen because chemotherapy attacks both your healthy cells as well as cancer cells.

Immunotherapy works differently. From the time you were born, your body has been producing cancer cells. Normally, your immune system sees these cancer cells and kills them off before they can grow. However, as you get older, the cancer cells get smarter and your immune system gets weaker. Cancer cells learn to "trick" your immune system into thinking that the cancer cells belong by masquerading cancer cells as normal, healthy tissue. Your immune system leaves the cancer cells alone, thinking that it is doing its job, while the cancer grows unchecked.

Immunotherapy works by revealing the cancer cells to your immune system. Your immune system realizes, *Hey, this is not supposed to be here,* and kills the cancer cells. With immunotherapy, we thus enable your body to do the job it was designed to do all along.

Because of this, side effects from immunotherapy are very different than side effects from chemotherapy. In essence, we are "revving" up your immune system. The side effects that you can experience from immunotherapy are similar to the side effects of having an overactive immune system. Patients can get fatigue, rash, joint pain, thyroid issues, and diarrhea. However, as a whole, immunotherapy tends to be very well-tolerated, and has provided powerful and amazing results for patients with certain types of cancers.

While immunotherapy has been revolutionary for the treatment of certain types of cancers, it is important to note that immunotherapy has not been approved or tested in all types or stages of cancer. For this reason, your medical oncologist may be unable to offer you immunotherapy outside the role of a **clinical trial**. In addition, some types of cancers do not respond well to immunotherapy. If studies have shown that immunotherapy does not result in shrinkage of your cancer type, your oncologist will recommend using a medication that will provide you with better results.

If you are interested in learning more about immunotherapy and whether it is an appropriate treatment for you, please discuss it further with your oncologist.

Chemoradiation

Although cancer cells are able to grow and replicate, ultimately, they are more fragile than normal, healthy cells. Radiation capitalizes on this fragility by adding stress to the cancer cells, causing them to die. Normal healthy cells grow back. Ideally, the cancer cells do not.

Sometimes, we add chemotherapy along with radiation to "boost" our radiation effects. This is known as "**concurrent chemoradiation**." Concurrent chemoradiation is typically used when a cancer is too large to cut out safely but still localized in one spot.

How does concurrent chemoradiation work? Imagine taking a hot bath at the end of the day. Typically, the heat of the water would feel relaxing and soothing. Now imagine taking that same hot bath with a sunburn. Instead of feeling soothing, the heat of the water now feels painful! What has changed? The temperature of the water is the same—the *sensitivity* of your skin has changed. Your sunburn has made your skin cells more sensitive to the water temperature.

Adding chemotherapy to radiation is like giving cancer cells a sunburn. Chemotherapy makes cancer cells more sensitive to radiation so that the same dose of radiation works more effectively.

MR. LARRY'S STORY

Mr. Larry was a 63-year-old man with newly diagnosed stage 3 lung cancer. His cancer was large and too close to his main airway to be surgically removed. In addition, multiple lymph nodes in his chest were biopsied and found to be positive for cancer. However, his scans showed no evidence of cancer outside of his lungs.

Given that there was a chance his cancer could be cured, I wanted to be aggressive with his treatment. However, at the same time, I knew that surgery would be impossible; there was no way to remove all his cancer and still leave him with normal functioning lungs. With that in mind, I recommended concurrent chemoradiation. He would receive IV chemotherapy weekly in conjunction with daily radiation. The chemotherapy would make his radiation work better, and the radiation would hopefully kill the areas of cancer in his chest.

He finished six weeks of concurrent chemoradiation, which he tolerated well. After finishing concurrent chemoradiation, I recommended adjuvant immunotherapy every two weeks for one year in an effort to kill any cancer cells that had leaked into the blood system.

Mr. Larry has since completed his one year of adjuvant immunotherapy. His most recent imaging shows no evidence of active cancer, and he is currently in remission.

Performance Status

"Performance status" is essentially a medical term for your overall well-being and robustness. Your performance status will guide many of our decisions regarding your cancer care, so it is an important concept to understand.

As mentioned already, chemotherapy has side effects. Often these side effects are unavoidable. However, your body has a certain level of reserve that will help you bounce back from these side effects. The more reserve you have, the easier it will be for you to recover from chemotherapy.

Imagine you were conducting a study on the effects of insomnia on the human body. You have two volunteers sign up for the study. Volunteer number one is a 20-year-old college student who is otherwise healthy. As per study protocol, he stays up for 48 hours straight with no sleep. At the end of those 48 hours, you check his vital signs, reflexes, and symptoms. While he is tired and cranky, he is otherwise fine. You let him go home, he crashes for 12 hours, and he wakes up feeling more or less his usual self.

Now imagine volunteer number two is a 65-year-old man who has just recovered from the flu. Again, as per study guidelines, he stays up for 48 hours. By the end of those 48 hours, however, he's coughing, barely able to stand, and starting to run a fever. He goes home, sleeps for eight hours, and ends up checking into the Emergency Department for dehydration.

Why did the two volunteers have different outcomes?

Some people might say age. As we get older, our ability to heal and recover from illness and injury gets slower. Even small insults to the body, such as sleep deprivation, can have a more profound impact on someone older compared to someone younger.

Other people may point out that volunteer number two was recovering from the flu. By depriving his body of sleep, he lost the opportunity to rest and recover his resources.

At the end of the day, both of these answers are right. Volunteer number two was more ill compared to volunteer number one due to having a lower *performance status*. As mentioned, performance status is a general sense of a person's overall well-being and robustness. If your body has already been weakened, whether by age or other medical issues, your ability to "bounce back" from an injury or stressor will be lower. Thus, it will take less injury or stress to result in harm, possibly even death.

Why is this important? Chemotherapy, surgery, and radiation are all stressors to the body. As a doctor, my first rule is, "Do no harm." I am treating you—all of you, not just your cancer. With that in mind, I use your performance status as a gauge of how much stress your body can handle. When considering your treatment options, I consider your performance status and the toxicity of my treatments. If the benefit of treatment does not outweigh the risks, I will not offer the treatment.

How is performance status judged? As an oncologist, I frequently use something known as the ECOG Scale of Performance Status. ECOG 0 is considered the best performance status, ECOG 5 is considered the worst.

Remember our 20-year-old college student with no other health issues? He has an ECOG of 0. He dresses himself and does all his own cooking, cleaning, and food shopping. He attends school full-time, works part-time, and goes to the gym regularly. He is fully active and able to do all his life activities normally.

Imagine that same college student has a head cold. He is feeling stuffy and congested, but he is still going to classes and able to take care of himself. He might skip the gym and go to bed early, but he's otherwise able to accomplish his normal activities. In this situation, he would have an ECOG of 1.

Now imagine that his head cold is getting worse. He's starting to have a cough and a low grade fever. While he can still feed and dress himself, he's taking naps throughout the day and skipping some classes and work shifts. At this time, he has an ECOG of 2.

Unfortunately, now our college student is sick as a dog. He has the full-blown flu, with headache, coughs, high fevers, and fatigue. He's spending all his time in bed, only getting out of bed for food, water and to go to the bathroom. All cooking, food shopping, and household chores have to be taken care of by his girlfriend. During this time, he has an ECOG of 3.

ECOG 4 implies an inability to carry out any self-care, and complete confinement to a bed or chair. If our college student was sick enough to the point that he could not even feed himself or go to the bathroom by himself, he would have had an ECOG of 4.

Finally, ECOG 5 implies death.

Grade	ECOG Performance Status
0	Fully active, able to carry on all pre-disease performance without restriction
1	Restricted in physically strenuous activity but ambulatory and able to carry out work of light or sedentary nature (e.g., light house work, office work)
2	Ambulatory and capable of all self-care but unable to carry out any work activities; up and about more than 50 percent of waking hours

3	Capable of only limited self-care; confined to bed or chair more than 50 percent of waking hours
4	Completely disabled; cannot carry on any self-care; totally confined to bed or chair
5	Death

ECOG performance status is an extremely useful way to gauge someone's robustness. If a patient tells me that she does her own cooking, cleaning, and grocery shopping, I know that she is fairly active and independent. Even if she is 87-years-old, she has enough mobility and reserve to tolerate treatment. Conversely, if I have a 57-year-old patient with heart failure, kidney failure, and severe diabetes, who mostly requires a wheelchair or scooter for transportation, I know that her reserve will be a lot less. I will have to be very careful about the treatment I provide, lest I actually harm her instead of help her.

Why is this important? Because *your* performance status will directly impact the cancer treatments your oncologist offers *you*. Often I will choose one chemotherapy regimen over another based on a patient's performance status. Sometimes I will lower my chemotherapy dose from the onset to ensure that my chemotherapy does not cause harm.

Even after you start your treatment, performance status continues to play a huge role in your care. At every appointment, I will assess your overall fitness and health. If you start having more fatigue, weakness, or weight loss, this suggests to me that your performance status is declining.

As your performance status declines, your ability to bounce back from your treatment declines, and I will need to adjust your chemotherapy accordingly.

How can you improve your performance status? You have probably heard the saying, "A body in motion stays in motion." This is true! Stay active. If you do not use it, you will lose it. Push yourself to get out of the chair even if you are tired. Walk to the mailbox. Walk around your house. Get out of bed and sit in a chair, and every time there is a commercial, walk a lap around your living room.

Secondly, eat. Try to hold on to your weight, and prevent the slow slide of weight loss. Weight loss during chemotherapy is not the same as regular weight loss—weight loss during chemotherapy is muscle loss. If you are able to, eat foods high in protein.[3] Protein builds muscle, and muscle is what keeps you active. When you start losing muscle, you start losing performance status.

Finally, stay engaged. Participate in life. Even if you cannot garden anymore, still go outside and sit on your porch. Even if you cannot go grocery shopping, help prepare dinner. The more you stay engaged with life, the more you will be inspired to keep active.

Prognosis

"Prognosis" is the term we use to characterize the likelihood your cancer will recur or the likelihood that you could

---

[3] Always clear changes in your diet with your doctor first.

die from your cancer. Other than the word "cancer" itself, prognosis can be one of the scariest words your doctor can mention. Some patients shy away from discussing prognosis, while other patients ask about it immediately.

How do I, as your oncologist, determine your prognosis? I determine your prognosis through a complicated algorithm that incorporates multiple factors. The most common basis for prognosis comes from the Surveillance, Epidemiology, and End Results program, known as the SEER program. The SEER program is a national collection of data regarding cancer incidence and survival from cancer registries across the country. Data regarding overall survival with different types of cancer can be found through the SEER program.

However, SEER data must be taken with a grain of salt. SEER data can date back ten, fifteen, even twenty years. So much has changed in oncology over the past twenty years that some of the data may actually be irrelevant.

In addition to SEER data, sometimes I use online calculators to determine prognosis. These calculators synthesize results from multiple studies and allow us to plug in details regarding your cancer size, number of positive lymph nodes, age, gender, and other factors to compute your prognosis. While these calculators can be extremely helpful, they are not available for every type of cancer. In addition, these calculators often do not take into account new treatment options and recent study findings.

With that in mind, I also use data from recent studies to determine your risk of recurrence and overall survival. If I am administering a treatment studied in a particular clinical trial, I will quote specific numbers from the clinical trial regarding the risk of cancer recurrence and patient overall survival.

Finally, I take your performance status into account. How healthy and robust you are determines what treatment options I can offer you, and how well you will tolerate the treatment side effects. No matter how large or aggressive your cancer might be, the better your performance status, the better your prognosis.

DR. DERIDDER'S STORY

Please do not try to calculate your own prognosis. It will be the first thing you will want to do after you hear the word "cancer." However, by relying on the internet instead of your doctor, you run the risk of exposing yourself to inaccurate information.

I was a patient in the Emergency Department myself once. I had come in with a facial droop, scared that I was having a stroke. The Emergency Department physician examined me and mentioned in passing a possible diagnosis of multiple sclerosis, also known as MS. As a physician, I knew a little bit about MS, and what I remembered from medical school was not optimistic.

Immediately after the physician left the room, I whipped out my phone and started Googling "multiple sclerosis." And I scared myself silly.

Waiting for my brain MRI in the Emergency Department that night, I ran through all the potential outcomes of being diagnosed with MS. I imagined being able to work and function, but having to deal with the strain of knowing my MS could flare up at any time. I imagined being debilitated, unable to work, and unable to provide for my family. I imagined myself dying, leaving my 2-year-old daughter without a mother.

An hour later, I was done with my brain MRI and the Emergency Department physician walked briskly into the room. "Your MRI looks fine," he said brightly. "I talked to the neurologist. You probably have Bell's palsy. You can go home. Your symptoms should go away in about a week." After giving me a prescription for steroids, he sent me home.

While it is human nature to want to understand and prepare yourself for the worst, do not subject yourself to the whims of the internet. Prognosis has far too many implications for your life to try and "guesstimate" it from the internet. I once had a patient come into my office sobbing, thinking that she was dying, when in fact her prognosis was excellent. "But on the internet, it said that I only had a 5 percent chance of being alive in five years," she said in disbelief.

"The internet must have been talking about a different type of cancer," I responded. "You are going to be fine."

While I do not recommend trying to figure out your own prognosis from the *internet*, I strongly recommend you talk to your *oncologist* about your prognosis. I think it is extremely important for you to understand the nature of your cancer. Only by being fully prepared and understanding your disease can you truly approach your situation.

What if you do not want to know your prognosis? I have had patients tell me, "I don't want to know the numbers." I have had patients say that they believe in the "power of positive thinking." "Dr. DeRidder," I've been told, "I'm not going to accept that my cancer could come back."

Only you can decide whether or not you wish to know your prognosis. Personally, I think that knowing your prognosis helps you make better decisions regarding your treatment. Understanding the nature of your cancer does not in any way make your cancer worst. At the end of the day, God has a plan for you, and nothing I say or tell you is going to change that plan. Ultimately, you may live another twenty or thirty years. Or you may live another six months. The important thing is to be *prepared*. Prepare for the worst, but hope and pray for the best. The last thing I ever want a patient to tell me is, "Dr. DeRidder if I had just known, I would have done this all differently."

WHAT YOU HAVE LEARNED IN THIS CHAPTER

Summary:

- There are four cancer stages. Your cancer treatment options depend on your cancer stage.
- Treatment options include surgery, radiation, chemotherapy, immunotherapy, or a combination of chemotherapy and radiation known as chemoradiation
- Performance status is a medical term for your overall health and robustness. Your cancer doctor will recommend a treatment plan for you based on your cancer stage and your performance status.
- Your prognosis is based on your cancer stage, performance status, and treatment.

In this chapter, you have learned the basics behind cancer staging and why it is so important. We have discussed the concepts behind surgery, radiation, and chemotherapy/immunotherapy, as well as why and when these treatment modalities are used. You have been introduced to the concept of performance status, and learned how your cancer doctor determines your prognosis—and why you should ask about it.

Now that you have been armed with the basics, you are ready to attend your initial consult appointment with your oncologist. At your appointment, you will learn more about your oncologist's plan for treating your cancer. In the beginning of this chapter, I stated that I typically have an "agenda" I cover with my patients at their initial appointment. In the appendix, you can find a copy of this agenda to bring with you to your appointment, with space for you to write your notes on the side.

If you have made it this far in your reading, congratulations! As I said in the beginning of this book, knowledge is power. The more prepared you are, the better equipped you will be to process the influx of information you will receive at your first oncology appointment.

In the next chapter, I will discuss how to prepare for some of the medical, social, and emotional aspects of your cancer consult appointment.

CHAPTER 2

Making the Most of Your Consult

"So, in summary, you have a stage 2 breast cancer, with cancer involving one of the lymph nodes. Because cancer is in the lymph node, I'd recommend you receive chemotherapy. We've reviewed the side effects and the next steps we would take if you want to move forward. What are your thoughts at this point?" I asked.

Ms. Elizabeth looked over at her husband, Gerry. "What do you think?"

Gerry shook his head. "It's not what I think, it's what you think!" he replied.

"I just don't know," she said. "It's all so overwhelming. I just can't seem to wrap my head around everything." She closed her eyes and rubbed her hand over her forehead. After a moment, she opened her eyes and pointed towards a small notebook in her husband's lap. "Didn't you have some questions you wanted to ask the doctor?" she asked him.

"Yes, but I think we answered most of them," he replied, looking his list up and down. "We talked about the stage, side effects, prognosis...Oh, here's one we didn't talk about. Do you think we should get a second opinion?"

Ms. Elizabeth looked at me apologetically. "It's not that we don't believe what you are saying. But one of my friends went up the road for her treatment and she recommended I get a second opinion there. Do you think I need a second opinion? Would they do anything differently?"

"That's a good question," I answered her. "I am completely fine with you getting a second opinion. However, there are some pros and cons to that decision."

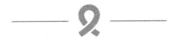

When you arrive for your initial oncology appointment, you will likely feel nervous and possibly overwhelmed. The medical, emotional, and social aspects of your appointment can be daunting. How do you prepare for your appointment? What questions should you ask? Whom should you bring with you? Like Ms. Elizabeth, you may feel overwhelmed by the information provided to you and the choices you will have to make.

The following chapter will discuss ways to prepare for your appointment, as well as how to prepare for the emotional as well as practical decisions you will need to consider *after* your appointment. Remember that you will have multiple opportunities to ask questions and learn about your diagnosis. Your cancer team is here to help you.

WHAT YOU WILL GET OUT OF THIS CHAPTER

Be prepared for your appointment	What information you should bring to your appointment.
What questions should I ask?	What questions to bring up during your appointment.
Whom to bring? Two's company...but three—four—five's a crowd	Whom to bring to your appointment.
Designate a point person	How to share information with family and friends.
Tell someone	Whom to tell about your appointment.
It is okay to switch doctors	What to do if you and your oncologist do not "click."
It is okay to get a second opinion	Whether or not you should get a second opinion.

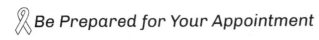

Be Prepared for Your Appointment

When you go for your initial consult appointment, you will likely need to spend between 10-15 minutes with the medical assistant or nurse doing something called "triage." Triage typically consists of checking your vital signs and going over your past medical history. Triage is a vital part of your oncology appointment. That being said, the less appointment time it takes to do triage, the more appointment time I have to discuss the important stuff—like your cancer treatment.

A little preparation goes a long way! Bring to your appointment a list of your medications, past medical history, past surgical history, and allergies. By coming prepared, you can maximize efficiency and make the most of your appointment time. Fill out the blank triage information list found in the appendix, make a copy of it, and hand a copy to the "triage" person at your oncology appointment. It will save everyone time, and ultimately, give *you* more time to spend with your doctor.

Below is an example of a triage information list.

Example Triage Information List	
Past medical history	1. High blood pressure 2. Sugar diabetes 3. Glaucoma 4. High cholesterol 5. Arthritis of left knee

Past surgical history	1. Removal of appendix – 1946 2. Removal of tonsils – 1949 3. Left knee replacement – 2010
Current medications	1. Amlodipine 10mg once a day 2. Metformin 500mg once a day 3. Carvedilol 25mg twice a day 4. Crestor 10mg once a day 5. Tylenol as needed for joint pain
Allergies	1. Penicillin – hives 2. Seasonal allergies
Social history (Marital status, occupation, smoking history, alcohol use, street drug use— heroin, cocaine, marijuana, etc.)	1. Married 2. Accountant – retired 3. Prior smoker – quit age 35 4. One beer once a week 5. No history of street drug use
Family history	1. Mother – died age 85, stroke 2. Father – died age 82, lung cancer 3. Brother – 55, alive, diabetes 4. Sister – 50, alive, breast cancer, diabetes 5. Son – age 34, no health issues

If you possess medical records pertaining to your cancer, such as biopsy or imaging results, you can certainly bring them to your oncology appointment with you. However, if you do not have access to these records, do not worry! The majority of the time whichever doctor referred you to my clinic will have already sent over the appropriate records.

If I find that I am missing something, I can usually get the information I need with a couple of phone calls.

Some labs and hospitals also offer online patient portals. If your doctor's office has an online patient portal that allows you to access your lab and imaging results, I would recommend enrolling. For instance, Labcorp has an online patient portal. After you register for an account, you gain access to labs you have had performed at Labcorp in the past. Likely your local imaging center, hospital, and oncology office have patient portals as well. I recommend asking about this feature, as patient portals can help you keep track of the testing you have had performed. By having your information at your fingertips, you can easily keep yourself, your family, and your doctors up to date and on the same page.[4]

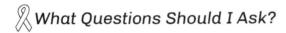

What Questions Should I Ask?

In my opinion, by the end of your appointment, you should have the answer to each of the questions listed below.

DR. DERIDDER'S QUESTION LIST
What type of cancer do I have (breast, lung, colon, bladder, etc.)?   What is my cancer stage?   What are my treatment options?   What are the treatment side effects?

[4] There may be a delay between having a test performed and having the results posted on your patient portal.

36

What is my prognosis (both with treatment and with-out any treatment)?

What do we need to accomplish before we can get started with treatment?

What is my anticipated start date?

In the appendix, you can find a copy of this agenda to bring with you to your appointment, with space for you to write your notes on the side. You can also find a number of web-sites online devoted to discussing the best questions to ask at your oncology appointment.

Hearing the answers to the questions above will help you develop a framework for your current situation. Before you can understand your future, you have to understand your present. Armed with this question list, you will be in a good place to move forward with your cancer care.

Whom to Bring? Two's Company...
but Three—Four—Five's a Crowd

Bring someone with you to your doctor's appointment. However, do not bring everyone.

MS. LAURA'S STORY

Ms. Laura was a 52-year-old woman with stage 4 breast cancer. She came to her initial consult ap-pointment in a wheelchair, due to back pain from cancer involving her spine. Accompanying her to her appointment were her three sisters, a cousin, her cousin's 9-year-old daughter, and the patient's mother. In total, there were eight people in the exam room, including her and myself.

Upon hearing Ms. Laura's diagnosis and prognosis, mayhem broke out in the exam room. Her mother, cousin, and the 9-year-old began crying. One sister got up and ran out of the room. "Go after her," Ms. Laura said. "She gets like this."

Following Ms. Laura's wishes, I left the exam room and found her sister sitting on the floor of the waiting room, crying and rocking back and forth. Other patients in the waiting room stared at her anxiously. "Please, ma'am," I said, trying to help her up off the floor. "We need to go back to your sister."

Ms. Laura's family members obviously cared about her. However, having multiple family members at her appointment drew focus away from why we were there in the first place—Ms. Laura. Instead of talking to my patient, I was talking to her sister in the waiting room. Instead of answering Ms. Laura's questions, I was answering her mother's questions. Instead of discussing with Ms. Laura how to improve her pain, I was left trying to improve her sister's distress.

I recommend that you bring no more than two people with you to your oncology appointments. One should be your

point person or **power of attorney** (more information about designating a point person can be found in the next section of this chapter). The other person can be a close friend, parent, spouse, or adult child. After your appointment, tell your point person who to inform about your oncology visit, so that he or she can share information with those closest to you, and people can still feel involved in your care. Remind yourself that you will likely have multiple visits with your cancer doctor. If you have multiple individuals express a desire to accompany you to your appointments, have family and friends take turns accompanying you to your visits. Tell your loved ones that your doctor's office has a two guest limit if you are anxious about offending loved ones.

Ultimately, if you decide to bring more than two people with you to your appointment, choose wisely. Bring people who are good listeners, and who you know will be emotionally capable of handling tough conversations.

Designate a Point Person

Designate a close friend or family member as your "point person." Your "point person" will be the individual who helps disseminate information to other family and friends.

While it can be affirming to have people inquire about the state of your health, if you have a very large family or group of friends, it can be exhausting to rehash your office visit or latest scan with every person in your network. A similar problem frequently happens to pregnant women. Friends, family, and co-workers all care about the woman and baby and want updates to assure themselves that everything is going smoothly. That's nice—up to a point. However, imagine you were going into labor. Would you want your mother-in-law, neighbor, and brother all peeking into the room while you are actively trying to have a baby? Most people would say no.

To solve this issue, nowadays, expecting mothers are encouraged to appoint a "point person," who will serve as a buffer between them and the outside world. The point person gives family and friends updates about office visits. When the expectant mother goes into labor, the point person stands at the bedside and gives encouragement. The point person also intermittently goes back out to the waiting room to give other friends and family updates on the situation. The point person thus serves the role of liaison between the patient and friends and family.

Similarly, while receiving your cancer treatment, many people may reach out to you. While some conversations may bring you peace or hope, others may drain you. Designate a point person, and discuss what role you would like your point person to play. You may want to have conversations with your family members directly, but have your point person filter information to your friends. You may want to have your point person serve as the point of contact for everyone. How much of a role you want your point person to play is completely up to you.

POINT PERSON, HEALTH CARE PROXY, AND POWER OF ATTORNEY.

I would like to clarify the difference between *point person*, **health care proxy**, and *power of attorney*. Your *point person* serves as a gatherer and disseminator of information. This is typically a verbal assignment. Your *health care proxy* is the person who is authorized to make medical decisions on your behalf in the event you are unable to make medical decisions on your own. You typically identify your health care proxy in a document called "**Advanced Directives**," also known as a "living will." Finally, your *power of attorney*, also known as POA, serves as a legal and financial decision maker for you in the event you are unable to make legal and financial decisions on your own. You identify this person in a legal document which requires witnesses and notarization.

Imagine if you were hospitalized and unable to make decisions for yourself. Your *point person* would be the person giving family and friends updates about your condition. Your *health care proxy* would be the person the doctor calls if a major medical decision needed to be discussed. Your *POA* would the person the hospital talks to about paying your medical bills.

Sometimes the role of a point person, health care proxy, and POA are all performed by one individual. This is ideal, as your point person often has been the closest witness to your cancer journey. However, sometimes your point person, health care proxy and POA are different individuals. I recommend that you clearly designate who is serving as your point person, health care proxy and POA (or if one individual will perform all these roles). Ambiguity in these situations can cause emotional and legal havoc for your family and loved ones. Clearly state your wishes and communicate these wishes to the people you have trusted with these special roles.

If you would like to learn more about POAs, health care proxies and advanced directives, the American Cancer Society has information available on their website. You can also ask your cancer center's social worker or case manager for information about filling out advanced directives and designating a health care proxy and POA. Finally, you can request a referral to your cancer center's palliative care team for help with completing advanced directives.

Tell Someone

What if you do not *want* anyone to accompany you to your appointment? What if you are a very private person and do not want others to know about your diagnosis?

I understand your concerns, and it is wise to be selective in who you tell as well as how many people you tell. Once the world knows that you have a cancer diagnosis, you will be the recipient of well-meaning advice from everyone from your grandmother to your niece to your mailman. It can be overwhelming and distracting, and many well-intentioned people will try to sell you on treatments that will not work or may have worked for a different stage or type of cancer.

However, after the word "cancer" leaves your doctor's mouth, your brain will temporarily shut down. You will likely miss some important information during your conversation with your doctor. This is completely normal and expected. For this reason, despite how you might feel about your privacy, I strongly recommend that you tell someone close to you about your cancer diagnosis. You will benefit immensely from having someone act as a second set of ears during your initial oncology consultation.

As mentioned earlier in this chapter, at your first oncology appointment your cancer doctor will most likely provide you with key information regarding your cancer and treatment options. Having a friend or family member at your side who can write this information down for you can be very helpful. In addition, after your oncology appointment, this person can serve as your "sounding board." You will likely have important decisions to make based off the information your cancer doctor provides you. Together, with your confidante, you can review the facts and decide how you wish to move forward. For these reasons, I recommend you tell someone about your cancer diagnosis, and, if possible, have someone accompany you to your oncology appointment.

If you are female and have been diagnosed with cancer, it may be especially difficult for you to share your diagnosis with your loved ones. Women tend to be the epicenter of their families. Many of my female patients act as caregivers for a sick child, husband, or parent while battling cancer themselves. As women, we are so used to taking care of others that it can be hard to step back and rely on other people to care for us. Because of this, it may be difficult for you to reach out to a family member or friend and share your burdens. *They have enough to worry about*, you may think. *They don't need me to add more problems.*

However, to care for others, you must first take care of yourself. If you have ever traveled by airplane, you will probably recall your flight attendant going over their "pre-flight" message. One point the flight attendant stresses is that if for any reason the oxygen masks spring down from the ceiling, secure *your* oxygen mask first before helping *someone else* with their mask. Why? If you run out of oxygen, you will pass out and end up unable to help anyone, including yourself. So take care of yourself. Reach out to a friend or family member. Tell someone about your diagnosis and get the support you need early on in your treatment.

MS. BETH'S STORY

Ms. Beth was a 50-year-old woman diagnosed with stage 3 hormone receptor positive breast cancer. She had complete removal of her right breast and was seen by myself for discussion about chemotherapy. From the first appointment, Ms. Beth was resistant to the idea of chemotherapy. "My husband is in his sixties and not in very good health," she told me when we first met. "I have to be able to take care of him."

I discussed with Ms. Beth that while I understood her concerns, she would strongly benefit from chemotherapy. Without chemotherapy, she had more than a 20 percent chance of dying from her cancer in her lifetime. The chemotherapy that she would receive would be tough, but it would reduce her chances of cancer recurrence by about half.

Ms. Beth refused to discuss her cancer with her husband. "He doesn't need to be bothered by all this," she told me. "He's got enough to deal with already."

We spent multiple appointments reviewing the benefits and risks of chemotherapy. I discussed with her that if she should die from her cancer, her husband would be left with no one to care for him. Wouldn't it be better to receive treatment now, and ensure she could be there for him in the long run? What would she advise a friend, or a sister, to do if the roles were reversed? Would she like to attend a breast cancer survivor group to hear other patients' experiences?

Ms. Beth rejected these suggestions and ultimately decided not to receive chemotherapy. She transferred her care to another practice, and to this day, I wonder how she is doing.

Deciding not to pursue chemotherapy is your right. However, sometimes fear of side effects, fear of the unknown, or fear of being a burden on others can influence your treatment decisions. Having someone by your side that you trust and can rely on can help you make these tough decisions. It is highly likely that the people in your life care about and love you. These people are waiting to have a chance to return your kindness. Give them a chance to reciprocate your generosity and time. Give the people you love an opportunity to grow by letting them care for you.

It is Okay to Switch Doctors

While I will discuss this topic in more detail in Chapter 5, I would like to bring up a few key points about this issue now. Every doctor has a different bedside manner and a different approach to cancer treatment. Some doctors are more aggressive with treatment, while others are more conservative. Though our chemotherapy regimens and standards of treatment are the same across the country, the practice of oncology leaves a lot of room for individual treatment style. Unfortunately, you may find that you and your doctor's style do not "click." You may feel like your doctor does not spend enough time with you, or does not answer your questions. You may feel that he or she does not have enough experience in your type of cancer. Sometimes it boils down to feeling more comfortable with a female doctor, or vice versa.

If you feel like you and your doctor do not "click" at first, my recommendation is to give it some time. Hearing bad news is hard, and it is natural to dislike or feel wary towards someone telling you difficult information. Maybe you and your doctor have different communication styles. The point is, this is very early on in your relationship with your doctor, and your relationship is likely to warm up as you get to know each other.

However, if, over time you still feel that you cannot trust your oncologist, or that you need to switch to a different oncologist, know that your oncologist is not going to be offended. We became doctors because we want to help people. Personally, if my bedside manner or way of practicing leaves you unsatisfied, I would much rather you switch to a different doctor than be unhappy under my care.

If you feel like you need to switch to another doctor, call your doctor's office and ask to speak to the office manager. Explain to the office manager why you are unhappy or uncomfortable. The majority of the time, if you explain why you wish to switch to another doctor, the office manager will work with you to try to remedy the issue. For instance, if your oncologist is always running late, the office manager may suggest scheduling your appointment as the first appointment of the day. If you have difficulty understanding your doctor, the office manager may remind your oncologist to speak clearly and slowly during your office visits.

If there truly is a matter that cannot be fixed with a simple solution, the office manager will assist with transitioning you to another oncologist in the practice.[5] With that in mind, be honest with the office manager about the issue that you have with your current doctor. By clarifying the source of your discomfort, the practice can match you with a doctor better suited to your situation.

⚭ It is Okay to Get a Second Opinion

As what is known as a "community oncologist," I practice in a small oncology group located in a semi-rural region. Often, I have patients come to their initial consult appointment wondering if they should get a second opinion at a major cancer center.

The answer to this question is complex. Most individuals gravitate towards seeing a cancer doctor at a community hospital or practice. Why? Convenience. The majority of Americans live in small to mid-sized towns and cities. For most people, community practices are simply more abundant and easier to access than major cancer centers, which are typically located in large, metropolitan areas.

When considering if a community oncology practice is right for you, it is important to note that some types of cancers are seen more commonly in the community than others.

---

[5] Please note that all oncology practices are different. While many practices allow patients to transfer to another oncologist in the office, some practices do not. If you find that your doctor's office does not allow transfer of care, you may have to decide if you can tolerate your current oncologist, or if you wish to transfer to a different oncology group.

Breast, colorectal, lung, and prostate cancers are seen frequently in the community. Therefore, it is highly likely that your local oncologist is familiar and comfortable with treating these cancers. To find a list of the most common cancers in the U.S., search online for the American Cancer Society's Cancer Statistic Center.

In my opinion, if you have been diagnosed with a "common" type of cancer, a second opinion at a major cancer center is typically optional. Can you seek a second opinion? Absolutely! If having an expert weigh in on your case will empower you and help you move forward with treatment— then please, go ahead and seek a second opinion. I want you to feel comfortable and confident with your care. That being said, a second opinion is not 100 percent necessary. I strongly believe that community oncologists like myself can provide you excellent care close to home.

Alternatively, some cancers are rare, or more complex than the norm. As a community oncologist, I may see a particular type of rare cancer once or twice in my lifetime. This can be problematic. If I have no prior experience with a certain type of chemotherapy, I may not know what to anticipate in regards to side effects. I may not know when to choose one regimen over another.

With that in mind, if you have been diagnosed with a rare or complex type of cancer, consider seeking care at a tertiary care hospital. A tertiary care hospital is one that is dedicated to sub-specialty care, such as oncology, trauma, orthopedic surgery, etc. Tertiary care cancer centers tend to have oncologists who specialize in specific cancer fields, such as myeloma, leukemia, etc. An oncologist at a tertiary cancer center may have spent his or her entire career treating one type of cancer and therefore is considered an "expert" in the field. If you have a rare or difficult to treat type of cancer, you may need this level of cancer expertise.

Like everything in medicine, you will need to weigh the benefits and risks of seeking this level of cancer care.

Tertiary Cancer Center		Community Cancer Center	
Pros	**Cons**	**Pros**	**Cons**
Expertise	Often requires travel, which in turn requires time and money	Convenient	Lack of expertise for rare or complex cancers
Many clinical trials	Large, difficult to navigate hospital campus	Easy parking	Lack of clinical trials
Abundance of resources	May take longer for you to obtain a consultation appointment	Easy to navigate	Lack of specialized resources
Access to expert in other fields (such as surgery, radiation oncology, pathology, etc.)	If you require hospitalization, you may be hospitalized at a local hospital that does not have access to all your records	Can treat common cancers as per national standards with FDA approved treatments	May lack experts in other fields (such as surgery, radiation oncology, pathology, etc.)

More advanced imaging		If you require hospitaliza-tion, often you can be admitted to same hos-pital where you receive your cancer treatment	
		May be quicker for you to obtain consultation appointment	

In some situations, patients *must* receive treatment at a tertiary cancer center as opposed to a community oncology practice. In other situations, patients with rare cancer can still be treated locally, though they may benefit from having a second opinion at a tertiary cancer center. The examples below highlight two complex cases with different outcomes.

MR. THOMAS'S STORY

Mr. Thomas was a 55-year-old man who presented to the Emergency Department with fatigue and weakness. In the Emergency Department, he was found to have abnormal blood counts. I was consulted to see him and performed a bone marrow biopsy. His bone marrow biopsy showed that he had acute lympho-cytic leukemia, also known as ALL.

Acute leukemia is an aggressive form of blood cancer that if left untreated, is 100 percent fatal. However, with the correct treatment, it remains potentially curable. At our oncology practice, we do not treat acute leukemias due to the fact that acute leukemias are rare, patients require intensive monitoring, and treatment often requires a multidisciplinary staff familiar with complications that can arise from leukemia. I recommended that Mr. Thomas be transferred to the nearest tertiary care center.

Mr. Thomas was reluctant to be transferred, as the closest tertiary care hospital was three hours away. He and his family lived locally, and he was their sole source of income.

I explained to Mr. Thomas that his type of cancer was rare, aggressive, and required highly special-ized services that could not be provided by our hos-pital. Ultimately, Mr. Thomas was transferred to a tertiary care hospital to begin inpatient treatment for his acute leukemia.

MS. LUCINDA'S STORY

Ms. Lucinda was a 32-year-old Hispanic woman. After missing her period for three months, she took a pregnancy test, which came back positive. A couple weeks later, she developed abdominal pain and bleeding. Concerned that she was having a miscarriage, she presented to the Emergency Department for evaluation. Eventually, after multiple scans and repeat blood work, she was discovered to not be pregnant after all. Instead, she was diagnosed with a rare type of cancer known as gestational trophoblastic neoplasia.

She came to her consult appointment with me with no prior knowledge of her diagnosis. She was Spanish speaking only and lacked insurance, transportation, and family support. Her primary concern was how soon she would be able to return to work. I had to tell her that not only did she have cancer; she also needed weekly chemotherapy for up to six months.

Given the rareness of her condition, I normally would have referred to Ms. Lucinda to our closest tertiary cancer center, which is a world-renowned hospital located approximately 3 hours away. However, she lacked insurance, transportation, and motivation to travel. Though no one in my practice, including myself, had ever treated her type of cancer before, we could still safely provide her chemotherapy. Therefore, after much consideration, she and I decided that we would treat her locally. We were nearby, could provide full financial assistance, and could provide free weekly transportation for her treatment to and from her home.

The examples above highlight that every situation is unique. Sometimes, patients with complex and rare cancers *must* be treated at tertiary care centers. Sometimes, patients with complex and rare cancers can be treated locally. Every patient and situation is different, and there is no right or wrong answer.

If you decide to seek care at a tertiary care hospital or are *required* to seek care at a tertiary hospital due to the complexity of your cancer, you may still benefit from having a "local" oncologist. Sometimes, community and tertiary care doctors are able to take a "partnership" approach. By seeing a doctor locally for treatment or supportive care, but periodically following up with an oncologist at a tertiary care center, you may be able to have the best of both worlds.

MS. CYNTHIA'S STORY

Ms. Cynthia was a 70-year-old woman with a history of multiple myeloma. She received a chemotherapy injection with myself every week, and came to clinic to see me once a month. In addition, she saw a myeloma expert every three months at a tertiary cancer center.

Ms. Cynthia's arrangement worked well for everyone. She was able to easily come back and forth to my clinic to receive her weekly injections. I monitored her monthly for side effects and checked her labs. At the same time, her outside oncologist followed her case from a distance. If there were any signs of disease progression, her outside oncologist would be able to smoothly guide our treatment decisions.

By following with me locally as well as following with an oncologist at a tertiary care center, Ms. Cynthia was able to get her treatment close to home, and still be under the care of a myeloma expert at a world-renowned cancer center. The arrangement benefited her because she was able to have the best of both worlds. The situation benefited me, as her local oncologist, because if her disease progressed, I could always fall back on the guidance and knowledge a myeloma expert.

For many people, this "partnership" approach is an arrangement that works well for everyone. However, if you are considering this approach, there are a couple of important points to remember.

First, you will need to see an oncologist at a tertiary care center, and you will need to *keep going back*. In other words, you will need to go for an initial consult appointment, and then, like Ms. Cynthia, have routine follow up with your "expert" oncologist to keep her up to date on how things are going with your care.

"But Dr. DeRidder," you say, "I don't want to have to drive three hours just to spend five minutes in the doctor's office. Can't you just email Dr. Expert and find out her thoughts?"

Unfortunately, the answer is no. If you want to have an expert oncologist at a tertiary cancer center provide advice on your case, that oncologist will need to consider you her patient. Seeing your expert oncologist once is not enough. You have to continue to follow up on a routine basis.

WHY DO I HAVE TO KEEP SEEING MY OTHER ONCOLOGIST?

Imagine this scenario. You are interested in putting a new roof on your house. You set up an appointment with a prominent contracting company known as "Company X." You meet with Company X and discuss putting a specific type of roof on your house. After you leave the office, you meet with another contracting company, "Company Y." Company Y can offer you the roofing job with a faster turn around and less cost, so you decide to move forward with Company Y.

Company Y starts the roofing project, but halfway through the job hits a complication. Unfortunately, the project manager does not know of any way to solve the issue. "Let's call Company X and see what the project manager there would do," you say. After all, Company X should be familiar with your project, right?

You call and you ask your question. Project manager for Company X gets on the phone. "I'm so sorry, sir," the manager says. "I can't provide you with any advice. We are not actively providing you services, so legally I can't advise you or another company what to do. If you want our services, please schedule an appointment and bring in photos and information about the issue."

Similarly, if you see an expert in consultation at a tertiary care center, and then decide to seek care at a community practice, you will not offend anyone. However, at the same time, you cannot expect the expert oncologist to continue providing advice about your cancer if you are not actively following up with her. She cannot provide recommendations regarding your care without having seen you recently. A lot can change within a couple of months—even within a couple of weeks. It would not be legally or ethically appropriate to expect a doctor to provide recommendations in this situation.

Now, let's imagine another scenario. Again, you are interested in putting a new roof on your house. However, you realize the job will be complicated due to needing a special type of shingle. You decide to hire a local roofing company, but ask them to consult with a national roofing company that specializes in using the specific type of shingle you need. You meet with both companies, everyone agrees on the project, and the project gets started. Throughout the process, you continue to meet with both parties.

Halfway through the project, the special shingle starts crumbling. Company Y says, "We don't know what to do, we typically don't use this shingle. Let's call Company X." Company X says, "Sure, no problem. If you follow these instructions, we can fix the shingle."

The difference between the two scenarios is that in the second scenario, the expert was consulted and *remained* involved in the process. Similarly, if you wish to have a working partnership between your community oncologist and an expert oncologist, both parties have to be involved and invested in your cancer treatment.

Another point to emphasize is that your community oncologist can only offer treatments that are **Federal Drug Administration** (FDA) approved and recommended by the **National Comprehensive Cancer Network** (NCCN) for your type and stage of cancer. If a drug is not approved by the FDA or recommended by the NCCN guidelines for your particular type and stage of cancer, there is a high likelihood that your insurance will not cover the medication. No insurance coverage = a large bill for you.

As a community oncologist, I am very familiar with the struggles surrounding insurance coverage and the astronomical co-pays that patients can sometimes face. My practice takes into account the efficacy and impact of a drug, as well as the financial toxicity of a treatment. For that reason, the medications I prescribe for cancer treatment are restricted to those that are FDA and NCCN guidelines approved for your particular stage and type of cancer.

Occasionally, oncologists at tertiary cancer centers may recommend treatments that are not yet FDA approved for certain types of cancers, or not yet part of the NCCN guidelines. This can make things difficult, as most insurance companies will not pay for the medication, leaving patients disappointed and frustrated. If you seek a second opinion at a tertiary cancer center, and your oncologist recommends a drug that lacks FDA or NCCN guideline approval, please know that there is a good chance that your insurance company will refuse to pay for the medication.

Sometimes, tertiary cancer centers are able to surpass this issue through clinical trials. A clinical trial is an experiment where we are learning whether a drug is safe and effective for a specific type of cancer. Some of these drugs are brand new, and others have been around for decades but are used for different types of cancer. The end result is the same—trying to find new and better ways to treat cancer.

Often, drugs administered through a clinical trial are given to participants for free. This can be a huge benefit of going to a tertiary cancer center, as they have *many* more clinical trials than community practices. If you participate in a clinical trial at a tertiary care center, you will likely need to receive all your chemotherapy/treatments at the tertiary care center. You can still see your community oncologist for hydration, blood work, and transfusions if needed. However, any administration of the study drug will need to be performed at the center running the clinical trial.

SOMETIMES THE BEST SECOND OPINION IS THE FIRST OPINION

Some people feel the need to have an "expert" opinion before moving forward with treatment. Everyone is different. If you know that you are the type of person who will need an "expert" opinion before deciding on treatment, please set up an appointment at a tertiary cancer center as soon as possible.

If you are able to obtain your appointment in a timely manner, consider scheduling the appointment at the tertiary care center *before* your appointment with a local oncologist. Trust is an essential part of your relationship with your oncologist. Ultimately, you have to trust your community oncologist to move forward with treatment. See an expert first, and then decide if you want to establish care locally as well. Otherwise, if you see your local oncologist first but do not want to move forward without an "expert" opinion, you may delay starting your cancer treatment.

Ultimately, the decision of whether to seek an expert opinion is completely up to you. Weigh the risks versus the benefits, and make a decision you can feel comfortable with. If you wish to seek a second opinion, let your oncologist know, and he or she can even assist with arranging a referral. You can ask for recommendations from family and friends, research online, or even ask your oncologist who he or she would recommend. Know that whatever decision you make, your oncologist will support you.

WHAT YOU HAVE LEARNED IN THIS CHAPTER

Summary:

- Bring to your consultation appointment basic information about your other health conditions and medications.
- Ask your cancer doctor about your cancer type, stage, treatment options and side effects, prognosis and treatment start date.
- Bring no more than two people to your consult appointment.
- It takes time to develop a relationship with your cancer doctor. However, if you feel you need to switch doctors, it's okay to do so.
- Feel free to get a second opinion.

In this chapter, you have learned how to prepare for your consult appointment, and what questions to ask while you are in the office. You have learned who to bring to your appointment, and how to disseminate information about your cancer and treatment via a point person. Finally, you have learned about some of the emotional and practical considerations that accompany your initial cancer consultation.

Remember that this is only your first visit and that it takes time to develop trust and a close physician-patient relationship. Know that if you did not get all your questions answered at your first appointment, you will have multiple opportunities to have your questions addressed. Your cancer team is here to support and help you during this overwhelming and difficult time.

At this point, you have met your oncologist, you have learned about your cancer, and you may have even decided to proceed with treatment. In the next chapter, I will review potential treatment side effects and ways to manage and prevent chemotherapy symptoms.

CHAPTER 3

Treatment Side Effects

"Hi, dear," I said. "How are you doing?"

"I'm okay," Ms. Elizabeth replied. "Just nervous. It's my first day of chemo."

"That's completely normal," I told her. "Did you pick up your home anti-nausea meds?"

"Yup. And your nurse practitioner went over everything with us, so I think we know what to do." She swallowed. "When do you think I'll start losing my hair?"

I gave her a sympathetic look. She had beautiful blond hair.

"Well, it's different for everyone," I said. "Typically patients lose their hair between their first and second cycle. First, you'll notice some tingling and maybe a burning sensation. Then, the hair will typically fall out. Once the hair comes out, the tingling and burning sensation will go away."

"Okay," she said. Her eyes began to fill up with tears. Frowning, she shook her head quickly. "It's fine, I'm fine, *really. It's just the anxiety of not knowing what the side effects will be like."*

"I understand," I told her. "The first cycle is the hardest because you don't know what to expect. But it gets easier after this—you'll have a better idea of how your body is going to respond to the chemo. And once we know what side effects you'll experience, it'll be easier to prevent them in the future."

She nodded and wiped her eyes. "I know," she said. "Alright. Let's do this."

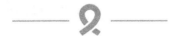

Many of my patients have had a family member or friend who has gone through chemotherapy in the past. "My mother received chemotherapy," my patient will tell me. "She was so sick. I don't ever want to go through that." Like Ms. Elizabeth, many patients fear the side effects of chemotherapy almost as much as they fear cancer itself.

Good news—chemotherapy and our methods of treating chemotherapy side effects have improved dramatically over the past ten to twenty years. While you will likely have *some* side effects from your treatment, ultimately the goal is to get you through chemotherapy as smoothly as possible. There will always be days that you will have less appetite and more fatigue than usual. However, the goal is to keep you as healthy as possible, and I will work with you to try to achieve that goal.

WHAT YOU WILL GET OUT OF THIS CHAPTER

Nausea	How to manage nausea.
Diarrhea	How to manage diarrhea.
Constipation	How to manage constipation.
Mucositis	How to manage mucositis.
Hair loss	What you need to know about hair loss.
Fever and neutropenic fever	What you need to know about fever.

Nausea

If you ask someone off the street about possible side effects of chemotherapy, nine times out of ten, that person would mention nausea. Unfortunately, nausea is a common side effect of almost every chemotherapy regimen. That being said, we have definitely gotten much better at preventing and treating nausea over the past couple of decades. In the following section, I will detail some methods to prevent and treat nausea.

Foods/Drinks

First and foremost, stay hydrated. Gatorade, Powerade, and Pedialyte are great options to use to replace electrolytes. If you find that your nausea is relieved with cold drinks, you can even make popsicles out of Gatorade using popsicle molds you purchase online. Ginger ale, flavored water, ice tea—all of these fluids, except coffee and energy drinks, count as hydration.

Bread, noodles, rice, potatoes, crackers, and even chips are food options that can help improve nausea. These foods are starchy and hold on to water, which can help settle your stomach. Soups and broths can provide fluid and help replace lost sodium. Ginger and mint can also be helpful to soothe your stomach. Both ginger and mint can be found as teas, candies, and drops, and will not interact with your chemotherapy. Eat small and frequent meals of whatever appeals to you. Remind yourself to eat something, but do not push yourself if you feel like you are going to be sick.

Medications

There are many medications for the prevention and treatment of nausea. Before taking any new medications, please discuss nausea management with your oncologist. Ask your oncologist how he or she recommends you prevent and control your nausea. In my practice, I frequently prescribe **Zofran**, also known as ondansetron, and **Compazine**, also known as prochlorperazine, for nausea control. Zofran is taken either 4mg or 8mg every eight hours for nausea, and Compazine is taken 10mg every six hours as needed for nausea. The two medications work in different methods, and for most patients can be taken together or interchangeably. The most common side effects of Zofran include constipation and headaches. The most common side effect of Compazine is drowsiness. I typically have patients try Zofran first, and if there is no relief of symptoms within thirty minutes, they can take Compazine.

With your first cycle of chemotherapy, it pays to be extra cautious, as you do not know how your body will react to your treatment. I typically tell my patients the following advice: The evening of your first day of chemotherapy, take Compazine before bedtime. Then, as soon as your feet hit the floor the following morning, start taking Zofran every eight hours for three days. During the next three days, take your Zofran regardless if you are experiencing nausea or not. It is always easier to *prevent* nausea than to get *rid* of nausea. You can take your Compazine as needed every six hours if you experience nausea that is not controlled with your Zofran, also known as "breakthrough nausea." Once you are about five days out from the day your chemotherapy was administered, as long as you are feeling well, you can scale back on your nausea medications and only use them as needed for symptoms.

The figure below highlights how I manage nausea for the majority of my patients (figure 2). Again, please discuss nausea prevention with your oncologist, and find out how he or she recommends that you take your nausea medications. Please remember that Zofran tends to cause constipation, so if you are taking Zofran around the clock, keep a close eye on the frequency of your bowel movements. If you are having less than one bowel movement per day, you may need to start taking a stool softener (more information about constipation can be found later in this chapter).

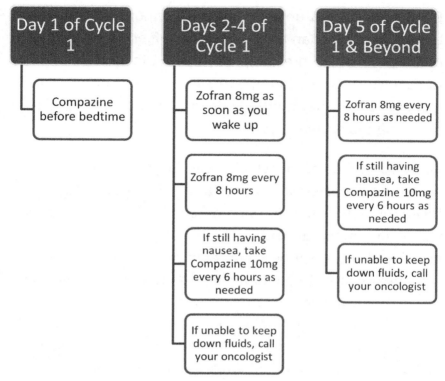

Figure 2: *Nausea management flow chart.*

If you have had no relief with Zofran and Compazine, your doctor may prescribe you other medications for nausea control. Alternative medications include **dexamethasone**, which is an oral steroid, **Phenergan**, a medication in the same family as Compazine, and even **Ativan**, which is an anti-anxiety medication that also has anti-nausea properties. If you have persistent nausea that lasts more than a week, your oncologist may consider prescribing something known as a **Sancuso patch**. A Sancuso patch is applied to the skin and worn for seven days, and works by releasing a long-acting form of anti-nausea medication.

IV hydration with anti-nausea medications administered through your IV can also be helpful. I frequently schedule patients to come in a couple of days after chemotherapy to receive IV hydration and possible IV anti-nausea medications. I find that a little hydration can go a long way in breaking the nausea cycle.

Finally, keep track of which days in your chemotherapy cycle you experience nausea. If you had nausea on days three through five after chemotherapy, anticipate that you will have nausea during the same period of your next cycle. These days will be your "high risk" nausea days. For your next cycle of chemotherapy, go ahead and take your anti-nausea medications around the clock on your "high risk" nausea days. Do not wait until you become nauseous to take your medications. Anticipate that you will have nausea during your "high risk" days, and start taking your medications empirically. After your "high risk" time period has passed, you can go back to taking your anti-nausea medications only as needed.

The important thing to remember is that there really is a *lot* we can do for nausea. The severe nausea and vomiting that patients used to experience with chemotherapy really is, for the most part, a thing of the past.

Diarrhea

According to the Infectious Diseases Society of America, diarrhea is defined as the "passage of loose or watery stools, typically at least three times in a 24 hour period."[6] Anything less than three times in a 24 hour period is considered "loose stools" rather than diarrhea.

The distinction between "loose stools" and "diarrhea" is a small but important difference. The symptoms that you describe to me ultimately affect how I approach your cancer treatment. As your cancer doctor, if you tell me that you are having diarrhea, I typically envision that you are having five to six bowel movements a day for multiple days. To me, that frequency of bowel movements is a serious impairment of quality of life, and I will likely alter your treatment based on your symptoms. However, if you were actually only having two loose stools a day, I may have adjusted your treatment unnecessarily. For that reason, it is important for all of us to be using the same terminology.

Regardless if you are having loose stools or diarrhea, there is a lot that we can do to improve your symptoms. Below, I will detail several ways you can potentially improve your diarrhea through both nutrition and medicine.

Foods/Drinks

First, hydration is key. As mentioned before, Gatorade, Powerade, and Pedialyte are great options to replace electrolytes. When it comes to food, treating diarrhea is

---

[6] 2017 Infectious Diseases Society of America Clinical Practice Guidelines for the Diagnosis and Management of Infectious Diarrhea. Shane AL, Mody RK, Crump JA, Tarr PI, Steiner TS, Kotloff K, Langley JM, Wanke C, Warren CA, Cheng AC, Cantey J, Pickering LK. Clin Infect Dis. 2017;65 (12):e45.

similar to treating nausea. Eating foods like oatmeal, cream of wheat, noodles, rice, potatoes, and crackers are food options that are starchy and help to absorb water. This, in turn, will make it harder for you to lose water through your stools. Bananas are also helpful because they have a lot of potassium, which people tend to lose with diarrhea. Soup and broths can also help replace lost sodium.

I would recommend avoiding dairy products if you are experiencing diarrhea or loose stools. The lining of your intestine contains an enzyme known as lactase. When you have multiple episodes of loose stool, the lining of the intestines is lost—and with it, all your lactase. Essentially, you become temporarily lactose intolerant. As anyone with lactose intolerance can attest, if you are lactose intolerant and you eat dairy, you are going to experience cramps, gas, and worsening diarrhea.

Medications

If you are still suffering from diarrhea despite the above measures, discuss your symptoms with your doctor. Describe what measures you have already taken, and ask your doctor if he or she thinks Imodium might help you. **Imodium**, also known as loperamide, is a medication that can be prescribed or picked up over the counter. Typically, the way Imodium is prescribed is that after your first episode of diarrhea for the day, you can take two pills. After that, you can take one pill after each *loose stool*, but no more than eight pills in a 24 hour period. If you find that you have taken the maximum dose of Imodium for more than two days, or if you are having a fever, severe belly pain, or blood in your stools, let your oncologist know immediately. Your cancer doctor may wish to do further testing.

The goal with Imodium is to keep the frequency of your bowel movements to less than twice a day, and to keep the consistency to that of soft-serve ice cream. With this in mind, it is okay to use Imodium as needed to achieve your desired bowel movement consistency and frequency. If you find that you have diarrhea every day unless you take one Imodium, go ahead and take one pill every day even before you have a loose stool. If you find that you have to take Imodium around the clock for the first three days after your chemotherapy, and then your bowels return to normal, that's okay. If you find that you need to take one Imodium every three days, that's okay, too! The key is to adjust your Imodium intake to achieve your desired bowel movement frequency and consistency.

MR. KEVIN'S STORY

Mr. Kevin was a 70-year-old man with stage 4 skin cancer that had spread to his lungs. He was doing great with his chemotherapy, except that his treatments caused him on and off diarrhea. I called him one day after he had missed his scheduled follow-up appointment with me.

"I'm so sorry, doc," he said over the phone. "I haven't been able to get out of the house. I get in the car and then I've got to go to the bathroom within a couple of miles."

"Have you been taking your Imodium?" I asked.

"Well, no," he said. "I took two pills after the first diarrhea, and then another pill after that. But then it made me constipated two days so I quit taking them."

"Why don't you take one pill after the first bowel movement?" I asked him. "Or take half a pill in the morning before you leave the house?"

There was a moment of silence over the phone. "I didn't know I could do that," he replied.

Mr. Kevin's lack of knowledge was not his fault—it was mine! As doctors, we often forget to tell patients that some medications are ok to titrate or to take as needed. As a patient, you are used to taking your medication exactly as prescribed on the bottle. However, diarrhea is one of those areas where there is a lot of flexibility with your medications, and it is typically okay for you to find what regimen works best for you. Remember to keep your oncologist informed about how you are taking your medications, but most doctors will let you find your own pace when it comes to diarrhea management. Remember—the key is titration. Your goal is to have one bowel movement a day.

If you are *still* having loose bowel movements despite taking Imodium, talk to your oncologist about a medication called **Lomotil**. Lomotil is a prescription drug that can help with diarrhea and can be taken in conjunction with Imodium. You can take it up to four times a day, and again, you can titrate your dose to achieve your desired stool consistency and frequency.

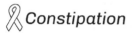 Constipation

Surprisingly, chemotherapy can cause constipation almost as frequently as diarrhea. Constipation can be difficult to deal with because it can sneak up on you. A day goes past without a bowel movement—no big deal, it will happen tomorrow, right? Then another day goes by, and then another day—and suddenly things are getting uncomfortable.

According to the American Gastroenterological Association guidelines, constipation is technically defined as "less than three bowel movements per week."[7] However, patients will often include other symptoms in their personal definition of constipation, including hard stool, feeling of incomplete evacuation, abdominal discomfort, bloating, and distention. Regardless if you are having one bowel movement per day or one bowel movement per week, if you are feeling blocked up, the end goal is the same—relief.

---

[7] American Gastroenterological Association. "American Gastroenterological Association Medical Position Statement on Constipation." Gastroenterology 2013;144:211-217.

Below, I will detail my approach to constipation in my practice. Please discuss with your oncologist before starting this regimen, as everyone is different, and what is safe for one person may not be safe for you.

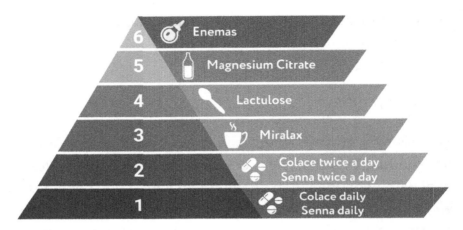

Figure 3: *The constipation management pyramid. Start with the recommendations at the bottom of the pyramid, and work your way to the top as needed.*

Colace (Docusate)

The gentlest medication that you can take for constipation is **Colace**, also known as docusate. Colace is a true stool softener, meaning that it works by making the stools softer. It will not increase your urge to go. Because it is so gentle, Colace typically takes 24 to 48 hours to be effective. Therefore, I usually tell my patients to start taking Colace daily from the start of their first cycle of chemotherapy. You can take it up to twice daily if you feel that your bowel movements are still too hard to pass. The goal is to have one bowel movement per day.

If you experience diarrhea with your chemotherapy, stop taking Colace until your bowel movements have gone back to once a day. If you experience more than 24 hours without a bowel movement, start taking the Colace again daily. Essentially, you are trying to calibrate your stool softeners with the goal of having one bowel movement per day.

Senna (Senakot)

If you are taking Colace daily and have still not achieved a daily bowel movement, add **senna**. Senna—also known as Senokot—is a laxative, meaning that it stimulates the intestines to move stool. It is available widely as a tablet and in some drug and grocery stores as a tea. It can take between 12 to 24 hours before senna becomes effective. If you remain constipated despite taking docusate and senna daily, you can take both medications twice a day.

Miralax

If you take Colace and senna twice a day for a couple of days and remain constipated, at that point I recommend adding **Miralax**. Miralax is an over the counter powder known as an osmotic. It draws water into the bowels, which helps to soften the stool and stimulate stool movement. Miralax typically takes 12 to 24 hours to be effective. Follow the instructions on the bottle to prepare it. Of note, to work best, it should be taken with 8 ounces of water.

Lactulose

At this point, if you are experiencing constipation, you should be taking Colace twice daily, senna twice daily, AND Miralax. If you are *still* having constipation despite using this regimen for a couple of days, ask your doctor to pre-scribe you **Lactulose**. Lactulose is a syrup that you can take up to four times a day. If you successfully have a bowel movement after adding Lactulose, you can likely cut back on the Miralax and senna, and just take lactulose in com-bination with docusate. Again, titration is key—your goal is to have one bowel movement a day. You may need to figure out what combination works best for your body.

Magnesium Citrate

If you have not had a bowel movement with the above reg-imen, you can take something called **magnesium citrate**. Magnesium citrate can be found at your local drug store or grocery store. It is a clear liquid that works as a pow-erful stimulant for constipation. If you have gone through the prior levels of the Constipation Pyramid (see figure 3) without having a bowel movement and are at the point that you feel this medication is necessary, please call your on-cologist first to confirm that it is appropriate for you to use. If your oncologist gives you the green light, take a third of a bottle (usually a bottle will be about 300ml, so take 100ml) mixed with an equal amount of water. If you have not had a bowel movement within four hours, take another third of the bottle with equal amounts of water. If you still have not had a bowel movement after another four hours, you can finish the bottle. Of note, this medication is a powerful laxative. Only take this if you are planning on being home for the next couple of hours, or you might have an embarrassing situation in your car or in public.

Enema

Up until now, we have been treating from the top down—everything has been oral. However, sometimes the problem is from below. If you have very hard, dry stool, it can literally form a ball inside your intestines. That ball can be so large that no matter what medications you take, the stool will not pass on its own.

If this is the case, you may need to use an **enema** or a suppository. Enemas and suppositories work from below and can both draw water into the intestines as well as stimulate the intestines. Again, please check with your oncologist before trying enemas or suppositories. For some patients, these may not be safe options.

If none of these interventions have worked, you need to go to the Emergency Department.

When administering chemotherapy, it can be impossible to predict who will develop constipation versus diarrhea. People who have a tendency to become constipated can suddenly have loose stools when starting chemotherapy and vice versa. I usually counsel patients that the first cycle of chemotherapy is a learning experience for all of us. Take notes! Your first cycle of chemotherapy will tell us what to expect from your body, and how to time your stool softeners to prevent constipation. Prevention is key—remember, by the time constipation hits, you are already two to three days behind. So if you have not had a bowel movement in 24 hours—start with Colace and go from there.

Mucositis

Mucositis is typically characterized as ulcers and irritation of the inside of the mouth and throat. Mucositis tends to occur between 5 to 10 days after chemotherapy and is more prominent with some forms of chemotherapy compared to others. While there is not a lot that you can do to prevent mucositis, there are a couple of things you can do to relieve it.

First, make sure that you actually have mucositis and not thrush. **Thrush** is a yeast infection of the mouth and throat, and can frequently occur when people are receiving chemotherapy. Get a spoon out of the kitchen and try gently scraping at a white spot in your mouth. If the white material scrapes off your mouth, you most likely have thrush. Call your oncologist, and he or she will give you a prescription for an anti-fungal medication that will clear the thrush up quickly.

However, if the white spots do not scrape off, you most likely have mucositis. First, stop using over-the-counter mouthwash. Over-the-counter mouthwash tends to contain astringent, such as peroxide, to kill bacteria. Astringents are great for killing bacteria but unfortunately can cause further damage to your already sensitive mucous membranes. Similarly, avoid using whitening toothpaste if you have mucositis, as whitening toothpaste can also contain hydrogen peroxide.

Instead, pour yourself a cup of warm water and mix in a ¼ of a teaspoon of baking soda and a ¼ of a teaspoon of salt in the water. Swish and spit a cup of this mixture around your mouth before and after each meal, and at bedtime. This mixture will help clean your mouth and prevent infection.

If your mouth remains sore, you can ask your doctor if he or she thinks you would benefit from "**Magic mouthwash**." Magic Mouthwash contains equal parts Benadryl, Maalox, and lidocaine. This mixture helps to neutralize the acid in your mouth as well as numb your mouth. Swish and spit your prescribed amount of Magic mouthwash before each meal. The solution will numb your mouth and hopefully make it slightly easier for you to eat. However, if you are still having trouble eating due to pain, let your oncologist know. He or she may need to prescribe you pain medications to take before eating so that you can keep up with your caloric needs. In addition to Magic Mouthwash, you can also take an over-the-counter supplement **L-Lysine**, which may help reduce the severity of your mucositis. During a mucositis outbreak, take L-Lysine 1000mg three times daily. You can subsequently take L-Lysine 500mg daily with your next cycle of chemotherapy in an attempt to prevent future mucositis flare-ups.

If your mucositis is severe, another medication that can sometimes help is a dexamethasone mouth rinse. Again, this would be prescribed by your oncologist. Dexamethasone mouth rinse is an oral steroid solution that can help calm down the inflammation in your mouth and promote healing. Typically, you swish and spit this medication several times a day as needed for mucositis. Of note, do not swallow this mixture unless otherwise instructed by your doctor.

Occasionally, patients who have had cold sores in the past will have an outbreak of something known as **gingivosto-matitis**, also referred to as Herpes Zoster or oral Shingles. This is a medical condition in which cold sores can oc-cur on your gums, tonsils, and the lining of your mouth. It can be extremely painful and typically requires treatment with a prescribed anti-viral medication known as **Valtrex**. If you are experiencing mucositis that is severe and does not seem to be improving despite using Magic Mouthwash, contact your oncologist for further evaluation.

Hair Loss

Hair loss does not happen with every type of chemotherapy. If you are concerned about potential chemotherapy-related hair loss, ask your oncologist what you should expect from your particular chemotherapy regimen.

If your oncologist tells you to expect to lose your hair, I'm sorry. Losing your hair, regardless of gender or age, can be extremely distressing. As a woman, I can empathize with the emotional and psychological distress that losing your hair may cause you. Unfortunately, there is not a lot that we can do to prevent hair loss. There has been some research using things like "cold caps" to help ameliorate hair loss. However, the cost of these products is high, the overall efficacy of these products is low, and they are not available at most cancer centers.

Typically, hair loss occurs towards the end of your first cycle/beginning of your second cycle of chemotherapy. First, you will notice a burning or sharp tingling on your scalp. This sensation happens because the hair follicles are being stunned by your chemotherapy. Once you experience this sensation, typically the hair will fall out soon after. Consider cutting your hair short or shaving your hair off at that time, as this can relieve some of the burning or tingling sensation since shorter hair tends to pull less at your scalp. The scalp pain will also completely resolve once the hair actually falls out.

Hair loss is never easy. It can affect your confidence. It may also be an uncomfortable symbol to others that you are undergoing chemotherapy. Many patients wear hats, beanies, or scarves during their cancer treatment. If you go online, you can find an abundance of tutorials for tying headscarves. You can also find many realistic wigs available online or at your local beauty store. If cost is of concern, ask your oncologist to refer you to your cancer center's social worker or case manager. Usually, your social worker or case manager will know of local organizations that offer free or discounted wigs, as well as have access to potential funds to help cover the cost of a wig.

Ask your case manager about support groups available in your local area. Support groups such as *Look Good, Feel Better*, can offer you a wonderful avenue to meet with other cancer patients, discuss how to manage side effects like hair loss, and develop relationships that will sustain you even after you complete your cancer treatment.

⚘ Fever and Neutropenic Fever

One of the most common—and potentially dangerous—side effects of chemotherapy is increased risk for infection. Infection can manifest in many ways, including fever. A body temperature measurement above 100.4 is considered a fever. If you are receiving chemotherapy and have a temperature greater than 100.4, call your oncologist.[8]

Imagine that it is 9pm. You are feeling tired but otherwise fine. You are about to go to bed, but you check your temperature because your oncologist instructed you to do so twice a day. Suddenly the thermometer flashes your temperature back at you. Surprisingly, it reads 100.5! You fish out your doctor's office number and prepare to call. As the on-call physician, what information will I want to know?

First, be prepared to tell me the name of your oncologist, the type of cancer you have, and, if you know the name, the chemotherapy regimen you are receiving.

Next, I will want to know the date of your last chemotherapy. Approximately 5 to 10 days after your last dose of chemotherapy is when your immune system is most suppressed. Your immune system is the barrier between you and the rest of the world. If your immune system disappears, the risk for infection is high. For this reason, if you tell me you

---

[8] Of note, some practices use 100.5 as the cut off.

received chemotherapy seven days ago, I am going to be much more cautious than if you tell me you received chemotherapy three weeks ago.

Next, if you can recall, tell me the last time you had labs performed. I will look at the labs and see what your white blood cell count was at that time (for more information about your white blood cell count, also known as WBC, go to Chapter 4). In the oncology field, our biggest concern is that your fever is a sign of infection. However, not all infections require hospitalization or even antibiotics. If your immune system is intact, your body will likely be able to fight off your infection on its own—meaning that there is a chance that you can stay home instead of having to come to the hospital.

Helpful Information to Have If Calling Your Doctor
Your name and date of birth
Your cancer doctor's name
Your cancer type
Your chemotherapy (if you know/can remember)
Last time you received chemotherapy (if you cannot remember the exact date, general time span is fine, i.e., one week ago, two weeks ago, etc.)
Your symptoms
Last time you had labs drawn

So, imagine you call me and tell me you received chemotherapy three weeks ago. You are running a temperature of 100.5, and you had labs performed yesterday. You are tired and have a slight sore throat, but you are otherwise fine. I check your labs, and I find that your WBC was normal yesterday morning.

Good news—you can most likely stay home.[9] Based on your labs and your symptoms, you most likely have a viral infection. Eat some soup, take some Tylenol, and I will have my nurse call you in the morning to check up on you. Though you may have an infection, your immune system is up and running, and you have an army prepared to fight and protect you. Sometimes, if you have symptoms suggesting a bacterial infection, your oncologist will call you in a prescription for antibiotics. However, the majority of patients with an intact immune system are fine to be treated for an infection without having to come to the hospital.

Now, imagine a different scenario. You have a fever of 100.5. You received treatment seven days ago. You had labs performed yesterday, and your WBC was 1.0, and your **absolute neutrophil count** (ANC) was 800 (to learn more about **neutropenia** and your ANC, turn to Chapter 4). You are not having any symptoms. Can you stay home?

Unfortunately, no. As mentioned, your immune system helps to form a barrier between you and the outside world. Interestingly, your immune system also causes you to have symptoms when you are sick. Symptoms of infection include chills, cough, runny nose, sore throat, diarrhea, belly pain,

---

[9] Remember, every patient is different, and only a healthcare provider from your cancer team is able to provide you with medical advice regarding your symptoms. If you are having a fever, please call your cancer doctor immediately for further recommendations.

or burning with urination. If you have an infection without an intact immune system, it is possible to have a severe infection with minimal symptoms. With a suppressed immune system, the only symptom of infection can be a fever. You could be on the verge of collapsing, and the only symptom would be a mild temperature.

This is the reason we, as oncologists, are so paranoid about fever. If you are neutropenic, fever may be the only red flag your body has available to let us know that something bad is occurring.

Now please, take a deep breath. I am not trying to cause panic. A fever is a manifestation of something else is going on in your body. The majority of the time, a fever itself is not dangerous.

MS. SUSAN'S STORY

Ms. Susan was a 34-year-old woman with stage 2 triple-negative breast cancer. She was receiving chemotherapy and had received her last dose of chemotherapy almost three weeks prior. She called the clinic at 11pm one evening, frantic.

"Dr. DeRidder, I just checked my temperature," she said hurriedly. "I have a temperature of 100.5. What should I do?"

I asked her the usual questions. When did you get your last chemotherapy, are you having any symptoms, etc. "No," she said. "I feel fine. Maybe a little runny nose, but my kids have had colds." She informed me that she was actually due to come into the clinic tomorrow for chemotherapy.

"Well," I told her, "let me pull up your chart and see what your labs have been doing with your chemotherapy. I'll call you right back."

"But...but I have a fever. Should I take Tylenol? I have a fever!" she exclaimed.

"It's ok, Ms. Susan. If you want to take Tylenol you can. But the fever itself is not what I'm worried about. Let me check into your labs and I'll call you right back."

I hung up and pulled up her chart. It appeared that her immune system had been holding up very well with chemotherapy. She had actually had labs performed earlier that morning that showed her WBC and ANC were normal.

I called Ms. Susan back. "Good news, Ms. Susan, you most likely have just a viral infection. Just stay hydrated and come in tomorrow for your appointment as scheduled."

"This is actually Susan's husband," a male voice responded. "Susan called 911 and is getting ready for the ambulance to come." Click. He had hung up.

Two hours later, I received a call from the Emergency Department. "Um, hi Dr. DeRidder," the ER doctor said. "We have a patient of one of your colleagues. She's here with a low-grade fever..."

I listened to the Emergency Department doctor tell me the same history Ms. Susan had told me. As expected, her WBC and ANC in the Emergency Department were normal. Her chest x-ray was normal and her urine test was normal.

"So...do you want me to do anything else?" he asked. "No," I said. "She can go home and come back to clinic tomorrow as scheduled for her appointment."

This is an example of what not to do. Please do not panic. Ms. Susan had the fear of neutropenic fever ingrained into her so deeply that her immediate response was to go the hospital. Unfortunately, all that the experience gained her was a hospital bill, missed sleep, and anxiety.

There are a couple key points to remember when it comes to fever in patients receiving chemotherapy. First, usually I am not concerned about the fever *itself*; I am concerned about whatever is *causing* the fever. Fever is a symptom. As an adult, unless your fever is greater than 103, the fever itself will not hurt you.

Second, my threshold for sending you to the Emergency Department depends on the date of your last chemotherapy, your WBC and ANC, and your symptoms. A fever in someone with an intact immune system does not always require hospitalization or a visit to the Emergency Department— however, your oncologist should be the one to make that determination.

Finally, neutropenic fever truly *is* an emergency. If you are neutropenic and have a fever, or there is a high suspicion that you are neutropenic and you have a fever, I will tell you to go to the Emergency Department. If your doctor tells you to go to the Emergency Department, please go. I have had people tell me, "Oh, I'll just keep monitoring my temperature, and if it gets worse I'll go." Or, "I'll just come to the clinic in the morning." With neutropenic fever, you might not be alive in the morning if you are not treated appropriately.

At the end of the day, it is better to be safe than sorry. If you have a temperature greater than 100.4, please call your oncology office. If it is during office hours, talk to the triage nurse. If it is after hours, speak to the on-call provider. Stay calm, and try to have details about your cancer and dates of chemotherapy ready. If your oncologist says you can stay home, take some Tylenol or Motrin, stay hydrated, and follow up with your oncologist if your symptoms get worse. If your oncologist says go to the Emergency Department, go to the Emergency Department.

WHAT YOU HAVE LEARNED IN THIS CHAPTER

Summary:

- If you are having nausea, the most important thing is to stay hydrated. Eat starchy, bland foods. Take your Zofran and Compazine. If you are still having nausea despite these measures, IV hydration from your oncologist can help.
- If you are having watery stools, determine if you are having "loose stools" or "diarrhea." Use the appropriate term when communicating with your doctor. Stay hydrated, eat starchy, bland foods. Take your Imodium and Lomotil.
- Constipation is very common during chemotherapy. Use the constipation pyramid. If more than 24 hours pass without having a bowel movement, work your way up the pyramid.
- Check your temperature according to your doctor's instructions. If you have a fever (some offices define this as a temperature of 100.4 or 100.5) **call your oncologist**.

In this chapter, you have learned how to manage the most common side effects of chemotherapy: nausea, diarrhea, constipation, mucositis, hair loss, and fever. While there are many other potential side effects of chemotherapy, the side effects I have discussed in this chapter are the ones that come up most often in my clinic. Fortunately, most of these side effects can be alleviated with both over the counter and prescription medications.

If you have additional questions about these side effects or questions about symptoms not discussed in this chapter, please talk to your oncologist.

In the next chapter, I will review common lab values that can be affected by your chemotherapy, as well as how these labs can affect your doctor's decisions regarding your treatment.

CHAPTER 4

Understanding Your Labs

Ms. Elizabeth was doing great with her chemotherapy. She had some nausea after her first cycle of chemotherapy but was able to manage it by taking her anti-nausea medications. I had scheduled her to return to the infusion center twice for IV hydration after her chemotherapy, which she reported helped significantly with her fatigue. We repeated this with cycle 2, and she seemed to breeze through her cycle without any hiccups.

She returned to clinic ready to receive cycle 3.

"How are you today?" I asked her. "From what my nurse tells me, it sounds like things have been going well since the last time we talked."

"That's about right," she replied. "I still get some nausea about two days after my chemo, but between the nausea meds and my hydration, it seems to be under control." She shrugged nonchalantly, and I had to smile. She had come so far from the scared, anxious patient of our first office visit.

"Well, I said, "I think, for the most part, you are doing terrific with your treatment." I pulled up her labs on the computer screen. I had reviewed them before entering the room, and I knew she was not going to like what I had to say next.

"However, looking at your labs," I told her, "your immune system is taking a bit of a beating from the chemotherapy. I expected this to happen, which is the reason you are getting a shot to boost up your immune system. However, despite the shot, your immune system is getting to be a little bit lower than I like it to be."

"So what does that mean?" she asked. "Is there something that I need to start eating, or start doing?"

"No, there's nothing that you need to start doing right now. It's all from the chemotherapy. I think we're okay to give you chemotherapy today, but we'll have to keep a close eye on things. If your immune system gets any lower in future, we might have to lower your dose of chemotherapy with your next cycle, or even hold your next cycle until your counts recover."

She looked at me with alarm. "You're going to lower my chemo? Is that safe?"

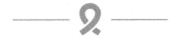

Once you start chemotherapy, you will hear your oncologist talk about your labs at each visit. In particular, we focus on your immune system, your red blood cell count, and your platelets. If you do not know what these terms mean, trust me, you are not alone. However, these labs directly influence your treatment, and like Ms. Elizabeth, you may find your treatment reduced or delayed if these labs return abnormal. If this happens, please don't panic! Mildly to moderately abnormal labs are very common during chemotherapy. For this reason, understanding these lab values and their importance will help you better anticipate and manage your cancer care.

With that in mind, the purpose of this chapter is to review some of the most important labs that can influence your treatment. I will focus mostly on your blood counts because, as mentioned, these labs typically have the greatest impact on your chemotherapy.

WHAT YOU WILL GET OUT OF THIS CHAPTER

Anemia	What anemia is and common causes of anemia.
Thrombocytopenia	What thrombocytopenia is and common causes of thrombocytopenia.
Neutropenia	What neutropenia is and why it is important.
Dose reductions	Why dose reductions are okay.

Anemia

Anemia is the condition of having low red blood cell levels, or **hemoglobin**, compared to normal parameters. Anemia typically occurs after you have received several cycles of chemotherapy. You may have symptoms from your anemia, such as fatigue, dizziness, or shortness of breath, or you may have no symptoms at all—everyone is different. Regardless, the treatment for anemia is the same. Your body needs more blood. How to achieve this goal depends on the cause of your anemia.

To understand anemia, imagine that each unit of blood is like a can of paint. You are standing in your local home improvement store, trying to buy a can. You approach the paint counter when you suddenly notice—the shelves are empty. The store has sold out of paint!

You go up to the counter and ask, "Why are there no cans left?"

The answer to this is simple. There is an imbalance between supply and demand, i.e, the amount of paint available on the shelves does not match the amount of paint needed. Interestingly, it turns out that your body's supply of blood is also a balance between supply and demand. Whenever this balance is disturbed, anemia can result.

But where is the imbalance occurring? How do we fix the problem?

Almost all your body's blood supply is produced by your **bone marrow**, the spongy tissue that resides in your hips and thighbones. Your bone marrow produces an incredibly large number of red blood cells each minute. Each red blood cell circulates in your body for about three months before it is recycled or destroyed by your **spleen**, the organ that sits under your left-sided rib cage. In almost all cases of anemia, there is imbalance between blood *production* and *destruction/loss*.

One common cause of anemia during chemotherapy is bone marrow suppression, or decreased *production*. Chemotherapy puts stress on the bone marrow, which in turn causes it to dial down production of new blood. Treatment of this anemia differs for each patient. In the majority of cases, anemia from chemotherapy is unrelated to nutrition, and diet and exercise will not significantly improve your blood production. However, if your oncologist states that you are also **iron deficient**, increasing your consumption of iron-rich foods may help improve your anemia. You can find information regarding iron-rich foods by searching online for foods high in iron.

Most of the time, your oncologist will simply observe your anemia, as it is an expected side effect of chemotherapy. However, if your anemia becomes severe enough, your oncologist may offer you a blood transfusion to replace the blood that your body is not producing. If this happens often, your oncologist will likely suggest reducing your dose of chemotherapy or holding your chemotherapy. Why? Chemotherapy is suppressing your bone marrow. If your oncologist does not back off on your chemotherapy, your anemia is only going to get worse. More information about chemotherapy **dose reductions** can be found later in this chapter.

Occasionally, your oncologist may be able to offer you a shot to help boost your blood production. However, there are special parameters that your oncologist must follow in order to administer this shot, and not every cancer patient qualifies for its safe administration.

Your body's production of blood is incredibly complex, and because of that, further discussion about the specific cause and treatment for anemia is beyond the scope of this book. However, if you have further questions about the cause of your anemia, I encourage you to bring them up with your oncologist.

Thrombocytopenia

You may have noticed in the past that if you cut yourself, you form a scab over the cut. That scab is made out of something called platelets. Platelets are tiny proteins that float around in your blood system. They stick together and help you stop bleeding.

Thrombocytopenia is the condition of having a low platelet count. Essentially, you do not have enough platelets floating around in your blood system, and when that happens, you can bleed more easily than normal.

Thrombocytopenia can occur for many different reasons during cancer and treatment. The same analogy that I used with blood production also applies to platelet production. In this case, imagine that platelets are plugs available at your local hardware store. In order for your hardware store to have plugs available on the shelves, there has to be the proper balance between supply from the factory and demand from consumers.

Your bone marrow makes your platelet supply and your spleen is responsible for recycling or destroying old platelets. If you develop thrombocytopenia, you have an imbalance between platelet *production* and *destruction/loss*.

Like anemia, the most common cause of thrombocytopenia during chemotherapy is suppression of the bone marrow or decreased *production*. As mentioned, chemotherapy puts stress on the bone marrow, which in turn causes the bone marrow to dial down production of new platelets. If your bone marrow is producing fewer platelets than usual but your spleen is still recycling platelets at its normal rate, you will end up with fewer platelets available. Like anemia, thrombocytopenia from chemotherapy is typically unrelated to nutrition, and diet and exercise will not significantly improve your platelet production.

The majority of the time, your oncologist will simply observe your thrombocytopenia, as it is an expected side effect of chemotherapy. However, if your thrombocytopenia becomes severe enough, your oncologist may offer you a platelet transfusion. Similar to anemia, if you require a platelet transfusion more than once, your oncologist will likely suggest reducing your dose of chemotherapy or holding your chemotherapy.

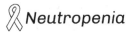Neutropenia

On a day-to-day basis, you most likely never think about your immune system. However, your immune system is constantly working in the background to protect you from infection.

Your immune system, also known as your **white blood cell count** (WBC), serves as both a fortress and an army. It initially serves as a barrier, trying to prevent bacteria and viruses from entering your body. If that fails, your immune system raises an army to fight off the invading organisms. You have two major armies at your disposal. You have a bacterial fighting army known as **neutrophils** and a viral fighting army known as **lymphocytes.** While both play important roles, your neutrophils are your A-team. Neutrophils protect you from all the bacteria out in the world trying to make you sick. In addition, they also protect you from all the bacteria *not* trying to make you sick.

Wait, what?

We all have bacteria that live 24/7 in our mouths, skin, and intestines. You have probably even heard of them before. The bacterium that lives symbiotically with our body is colloquially known as "good bacteria." You have "good bacteria" that live in your gut and help you digest your food, as well as "good bacteria" in your mouth and on your skin.

Good bacteria serve a purpose, and normally, because of your immune system, we all live in a happy balance together.

Chemotherapy often suppresses your bone marrow. When that happens, the factory that produces your immune system shuts down, your WBC drops and you become **neutropenic**. I typically consider people neutropenic when their total number of neutrophils, known as the *absolute neutrophil count* (ANC), is less than 1000.

If you are neutropenic, all the good bacteria that typically live in harmony with your body are given free rein to grow and conquer. With no immune system to keep them in check, the bacteria can grow—and grow—and grow. Suddenly the bacteria can show up in places where it is not supposed to and cause infection in your body. For this reason, if you are neutropenic, you will be advised to avoid activities that can lead to cuts and scrapes.

When you become neutropenic, you are also more susceptible to all the bacteria in your environment. Bacteria that your body previously would have wiped out in a matter of minutes now can set up shop and cause problems. That is where the concept of **neutropenic precautions** comes in. If your ANC is less than 1000, you will be instructed to use neutropenic precautions. This means scrupulous attention to handwashing. You will be cautioned to stay home as much as possible and avoid going out in crowds, where people can sneeze and cough and wheeze on you. You will need to time essential excursions to less busy parts of the day. If you are going to be in a room with more than 10 people, you may need to wear a mask that covers your nose and mouth to prevent breathing in someone else's germs.

Neutropenic precautions extend to food as well. While we may be used to thinking of fresh fruits and vegetables as nutritious and healthy, I caution my patients to avoid raw produce unless it has a removable skin. All of our raw, fresh produce comes from nature, and nature is *covered* in germs. With that in mind, my recommendations when it comes to produce are to peel it, cook it, or avoid it.

If you are neutropenic, you may need to avoid eating at restaurants, especially buffets or delis. First, restaurants tend to be crowded, and when you are neutropenic you should be avoiding crowds. In addition, when you go to a restaurant, there is no way for you to know how long your food has been sitting outside of the refrigerator, or how thoroughly your food was washed or cooked. While this would normally not be an issue for you and your healthy immune system, when you are neutropenic, this can be a recipe for disaster.

Most patients do *not* experience significant neutropenia with chemotherapy, and can still do the majority of their normal life activities while exercising caution. Discuss with your oncologist the likelihood you will develop neutropenia, and the level of precautions he or she recommends you exert. If your oncologist tells you that you are at high risk for neutropenia, remember, neutropenia does not last forever. Typically, neutropenia occurs around 7-10 days after chemotherapy. Once your ANC is greater than 1000, your immune system is back online and able to protect you, and you can likely resume most of your normal activities.

Given the seriousness of neutropenia, you may feel worried about experiencing neutropenia during your chemotherapy cycle. "Dr. DeRidder," you ask, "Is there something you can do to prevent neutropenia?"

Actually yes, there is something. It is called **Neulasta**."[10]

Neulasta is an injection that stimulates the growth of new neutrophils. Essentially, it is a chemical that tells your bone marrow to make and release new neutrophils ASAP. It is a wonderful medication that has saved thousands of lives. So what's the catch? Why not give Neulasta to everyone?

Your bone marrow lives in your bones, specifically, the long bones in your hips and your lower back. Neulasta works by telling the bone marrow to go on overdrive. Because Neulasta pushes the bone marrow to work harder, the biggest side effect of Neulasta is bone pain. For this reason, we give Neulasta only if you are at high risk of experiencing neutropenia with your chemotherapy regimen.

For some reason, taking Claritin the day before, the day of, and three days after receiving Neulasta can sometimes help relieve the bone pain. However, if Claritin does not provide enough relief, you may need to ask your oncologist for pain medications to help relieve some of the soreness.

---

[10] Neulasta also comes as biosimilar drugs Udenyca and Fulphila.

Of note, Neulasta comes as two versions—a shot and a patch. Both need to be administered between 24 to 72 hours after your chemotherapy dose. Occasionally, I will also use something called **Neupogen**.[11] Five doses of Neupogen = one of Neulasta. Each dose of Neupogen is much gentler than Neulasta because each dose of Neupogen is not as strong as Neulasta. Neupogen can be a good option in patients who have severe side effects from Neulasta. Remember, it is not as strong as Neulasta, so it is not as effective. However, if you simply cannot tolerate Neulasta, Neupogen may be used by your oncologist to help maintain your immune system with hopefully fewer side effects.

At the end of the day, remember, these medications save lives. Infection from neutropenia is a real and serious issue. While the lifestyle restrictions from neutropenic precautions and the side effects from Neulasta may be a pain— often literally—the goal is to keep you healthy and safe.

Dose Reductions

Your lab results and the side effects that you experience with your chemotherapy all serve as a guide map for how your body is reacting to your treatment. I use these markers, along with others, to help me measure how you are doing as a patient. Occasionally, I will need to adjust your chemotherapy based on the feedback your body is providing me.

---

[11] Neupogen also comes as biosimilar drugs Zarxio, Granix, and Nivestym.

The majority of the time, I initially prescribe a chemotherapy regimen exactly as it was administered in the original clinical trial that led to the medication's approval. As time goes on, however, occasionally I have to do something known as a "dose reduction." A dose reduction is when I lower a patient's dose of chemotherapy *below* the dose recommended by the FDA for a specific cancer treatment. For instance, if the recommended dose of paclitaxel for treating breast cancer is $80mg/m^2$, I will administer to my patient a dose of paclitaxel $60mg/m^2$.

Why would I lower a patient's chemotherapy dose? Well, as you know, all chemotherapy has side effects. All decisions regarding your treatment have to take these side effects into account. If the number and severity of your chemotherapy side effects begin to outweigh the potential benefits of your treatment, I need to adjust your treatment.

Often, patients are concerned that by lowering the dose of chemotherapy, we will reduce the efficacy of the medication. This is a valid concern. However, cancer treatment is not a one size fits all process. A dose of medication that might be right for someone else might be too strong for you.

Imagine meeting up with a friend for a cup of coffee. Your friend orders an extra-large dark roast with a shot of espresso. "I need my morning cup of coffee or I just can't get my day started," she explains. You decide to order the same thing.

An hour later, she's feeling great and ready to start her day. You, on the other hand, are feeling jittery, your heart is pounding, and you feel on edge. Why? The dose of caffeine was the same in both cups. However, the difference lies in how each of your bodies processed the caffeine. Your body required a lower dose of caffeine to feel alert. Anything above that dose manifested as unwanted side effects, such as jitteriness, anxiety, and palpitations.

Similarly, people can react differently to the same dose of chemotherapy. As an oncologist, my job is to take into account your medical history and your performance status to determine the safest dose of chemotherapy for you. After we administer your chemotherapy, my job is to adjust the dose for your next chemotherapy cycle based on the feedback your body is providing.

Unfortunately, I cannot tell you exactly how changing the dose of your treatment will ultimately affect your cancer outcome. However, my first rule as a doctor is "Do no harm." If my dose of chemotherapy is threatening to cause you significant and possibly permanent side effects, it is my duty to adjust your chemotherapy dose as needed. I want to give you the best cancer treatment possible. I do not want to risk permanently injuring you in the process!

MR. CLAYTON'S STORY

Mr. Clayton was a 65-year-old man with stage 4 colon cancer with a single site of metastases to his liver. He was otherwise very healthy and had a good performance status. The plan was for him to receive four cycles of neoadjuvant chemotherapy, and then undergo partial liver resection to remove the area of cancer.

From the start of Mr. Clayton's first cycle of chemotherapy, he had multiple side effects, ranging from nausea to severe chest pain requiring hospital admission. During his second cycle of chemotherapy, he became neutropenic despite receiving Neulasta. His neutropenia required us pushing back his third cycle of chemotherapy by two weeks to allow his bone marrow time to recover.

Given his profound side effects with his first two cycles of chemotherapy, I elected to reduce the dose of his chemotherapy medications with his third cycle. Mr. Clayton was concerned about the possible impact on his treatment's efficacy but understood my rationale for lowering his chemotherapy dose.

"I would rather you give me a lower dose of chemotherapy and keep me healthy," he told me, "than not be able to give me any chemotherapy at all because I'm too sick."

With that in mind, I lowered his dose of chemotherapy by 20 percent. He tolerated his third dose of chemotherapy significantly better than he had tolerated his prior cycles. Returning to clinic two weeks later, he looked better than he had since the day we started his cancer treatment.

He went on to complete his four planned cycles of neoadjuvant chemotherapy, with a significant amount of shrinkage of his liver metastases. He subsequently underwent resection of part of his liver and completed an additional eight cycles of adjuvant chemotherapy. He is currently one year out from his treatment, with no evidence of recurrent cancer on his most recent scan.

In the end, I would like to keep you on your original treatment as much as possible. However, if trouble arises, I will adjust your dose of chemotherapy to keep you healthy and get you through your chemotherapy safely.

WHAT YOU HAVE LEARNED IN THIS CHAPTER

Summary:

- Anemia is the condition of having low red blood cell levels. The most common cause of anemia during chemotherapy is decreased production by the bone marrow.
- Thrombocytopenia is the condition of having low platelet levels.
- Neutropenia is the condition of having a low immune system. If your absolute neutrophil count (ANC) is < 1000, you will need to use special precautions known as neutropenic precautions. If you develop

a fever when your ANC is <1000, this is a medical emergency and you should call your oncologist.

- Your oncologist may reduce your chemotherapy to prevent or treat anemia, thrombocytopenia or neutropenia. While a dose reduction could impact the efficacy of your chemotherapy, the ultimate goal is to keep you healthy.

In this chapter, I have reviewed three of the most important labs—your red blood cell count, platelets, and white blood cell count—that can affect your chemotherapy treatment, as well as the rationale for dose reductions. Please remember that everyone is different, and the dose that works well for one person may be too harsh for another person. More chemotherapy does not necessary equal better results.

At this point, you have started treatment, you have learned to manage your side effects, and you now understand commonly tested lab values and how they can influence your treatment. Now, we will start to explore how chemotherapy and living with cancer can affect other aspects of your life. In the next chapter, I will discuss how chemotherapy can affect your mental, emotional, and physical health.

CHAPTER 5

Living With Chemotherapy

"Good morning," I greeted Ms. Elizabeth. "How are you doing today?"

She had just completed 4 cycles of every other week chemotherapy, and was now about to start taking a gentler form of chemotherapy for 12 weeks. Today, she came to her appointment accompanied by her 20-something-year-old daughter.

"Tired," she replied. "That last cycle really took it out of me."
She paused. "So the next twelve treatments are typically easier?"

"Yes, typically," I told her. "Everyone is different of course, but I've had some patients even return to work during this part of treatment. You aren't going to be 100 percent, but usually, the side effects are not as bad as with your prior chemo."

"That would be great." She laughed. "Though I think I have gotten pretty good at managing the side effects."

"I think you've been doing a fantastic job," I reassured her. "You are doing exactly what you need to do—taking your medications, and taking it one day at a time."

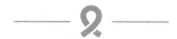

In this chapter, I will discuss living with chemotherapy. As part of this chapter, I will explore the growing relationship between you and your cancer doctor. I will also discuss the impact chemotherapy may have on your mental, emotional, and physical health. The goal of this chapter is to bring to light some common issues patients struggle with during their cancer treatment so that you are fully prepared for what lies ahead.

This chapter is broken down into four different segments, with each segment discussing a different aspect of living with chemotherapy.

WHAT YOU WILL GET OUT OF THIS CHAPTER

Part 1: You and your cancer doctor	How to improve communication with your doctor, and what to do if you and your doctor do not "click."
Part 2: Your mental, emotional and financial health during chemotherapy	How to adjust to life with chemotherapy and its mental, emotional, and financial side effects.

Part 3: Your physical health during chemotherapy	How to optimize your health during chemotherapy, including a discussion about diet, supplements, and complementary medicine
Part 4: Hospitalizations	Why your diagnosis and treatment may seem to change on a daily basis while in the hospital, and a reminder that medicine is both an art and a science.

Please remember that this book is written from the perspective of a cancer doctor, not a cancer survivor. There are many books written by cancer survivors that will detail their emotional journey through cancer diagnosis and treatment. The issues I address in the following chapter are questions I commonly encounter in my clinic, and the answers I most often provide to my patients. The goal of this book is to provide for you, as a patient, information that may not be available from other resources.

You and Your Cancer Doctor

"You were right," Ms. Elizabeth said with a smile. She had just completed 2 weeks of her "gentler" chemotherapy and had 10 more weeks to go. "I'm feeling pretty good. That first week I was still kind of dragging, but I think I'm starting to get better. I took a walk with my husband last night around the neighborhood and we didn't have to stop for any breaks. For me, that was huge."

"I'm so happy to hear that!" I told her. "Well, your labs also look great, so I think you're fine to receive your treatment tomorrow."

"Sounds good," she said. We chatted for a couple of minutes about how summer was ending too quickly, and she informed me that her daughter was leaving the following week to start her senior year in college.

I stood up to conclude the visit and walked toward the exam room door. As I started to turn the handle, I heard her say,

"Um, I did want to talk to you about one thing, though, if you have a moment."

"Okay." I turned around.

"One of my friends was recently diagnosed with colon cancer. It's a really tough situation..." She shook her head. "I don't know all the details, but she's being treated by a doctor at a different hospital. I happened to bump into her the other day and she told me that she hasn't been super happy with her doctor there. We got to talking, and I told her how well I've been doing. She told me that she'd liked to see you if possible. Is that something she could do?"

"I'm really sorry to hear that she's having such a tough time," I told her. "I'd be happy to see her. I'll give you our office manager's number, and your friend can call us to schedule an appointment."

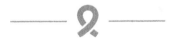

Unfortunately, Ms. Elizabeth's friend is not the first patient to struggle with the doctor-patient relationship. The relationship between a doctor and a patient is a unique and complicated one. In most relationships in life, it is a given that it will take time to build trust and understanding. However, often we expect patients to trust and respect their doctors after less than an hour's worth of conversation.

Ultimately, communication is key. By learning how to effectively communicate with your oncologist, you will develop a strong relationship together, which in turn will allow you to have your needs addressed in an appropriate manner. In the following section, I will review the skills you can use to ensure your doctor hears your complaints and answers your questions.

WHAT YOU WILL GET OUT OF THIS SECTION

Learn the difference between complaining and reporting	How to communicate side effects to your doctor.
Define your agenda	How to make sure your most important questions are answered.
It is okay to switch cancer doctors	What to do if you and your doctor do not "click."
Continue to see your primary care doctor (PCP)	Why it is important to continue to see your PCP.
Be nice	How to show your cancer team you appreciate their care.

℞ Learn the Difference between Reporting and Complaining

If you and your doctor have decided that chemotherapy is the right choice for you, you will likely have a visit known as a "chemotherapy education" prior to starting treatment. At this appointment, a nurse will go over with you a long list of potential side effects from your chemotherapy. General malaise, nausea, fatigue, constipation, and diarrhea are all very common side effects from treatment. Often these side effects are mild and will resolve on their own (see Chapter 3 for more information about chemotherapy side effects). However, some side effects may be important to let your cancer doctor know about, even if they are mild. So which side effects should you mention to your doctor at your next visit?

In my practice, my nurse rooms my patients. She reviews their vitals and medications and then asks them if they are experiencing any new symptoms. She then comes to my office to give me a quick synopsis. After we talk, I ask her, "Is the patient *reporting* these symptoms to me, or is the patient actually *complaining* about them?"

I find this method of categorizing symptoms extremely helpful. To me, if you are *reporting* a particular side effect, the side effect is mild and tolerable. Your goal with reporting a side effect is to make sure that as your cancer doctor, I am aware of what is going on with your health. If there is something that I can do to make the side effect better, you would of course appreciate it. However, overall the symptom is minor.

When you *complain* about a side effect, that particular side effect is bothersome and persistent. It is impacting your quality of life. You are making me aware because you cannot continue to live with that particular symptom.

Categorizing your symptoms can help you communicate with your doctor. It will help your oncologist know which symptoms to focus on during your appointment, while at the same time keep your doctor in the loop about all your symptoms.

MR. LINDON'S STORY

Mr. Lindon was a 75-year-old man with stage 3 esophageal cancer receiving potentially curative chemotherapy. His wife, who was his caregiver, was very anxious about him receiving treatment. While attending Mr. Lindon's chemotherapy education session, his wife requested a list of all potential side effects that Mr. Lindon could possibly experience from his chemotherapy.

Shortly after his first cycle of chemotherapy, Mr. Lindon returned to clinic for a follow up appointment. As I sat down in front of my computer, I smiled at him and his wife. "How are you doing?" I asked. I had already reviewed his labs, which for the most part looked within normal limits. His weight was stable compared to his prior visit. Both of these parameters suggested to me that overall, he was doing fairly well.

Mr. Lindon's wife took out a piece of crumpled paper. Of the 23 potential chemotherapy side effects listed, she had checked off almost all. "These are the side effects he experienced," she said, handing me the list.

Forty minutes later, I concluded that Mr. Lindon actually did very well during his first cycle of chemotherapy. He had some mild nausea, relieved by his home oral anti-nausea medications. He had some fatigue, as well as some intermittent loose stools, but both of these had improved. The only real issue that was still bothering him was persistent mouth sores. For his mucositis, I prescribed him a numbing oral solution and counseled him about using a baking soda mouth rinse after eating. Quickly, I scheduled him for his next chemotherapy cycle and concluded the visit. As I walked to the door, his wife exclaimed, "Oh, I had a couple of other questions about his chemotherapy I wanted to talk about!"

My conversation with the Lindons was an example of provider information overload. Mr. Lindon's wife had been told at her chemotherapy education appointment to "tell your doctor if you are having any of these symptoms." So, like a good caregiver, she was telling me about his side effects. The problem was on my end—I did not know which side effects were minor and which side effects we had to discuss in more detail. I spent the majority of his visit focusing on tolerable and minor symptoms, and ended up running out of time to address questions that actually mattered to him.

To help prevent provider information overload, I recommend you make a list of side effects that you experience. Then, divide your symptoms into two different categories. "Can live with/Improved on its own" and "Can't live with/ Still ongoing." Below, you'll see an example of what Mr. Lindon's list would have looked like.

Can Live with/Improved on Its Own	Can't Live with/Still Ongoing!
Nausea – intermittent the day after chemo, then gets better	Sores in my mouth – Painful, can't eat
Loose stool – about three days after chemo, then gets better	
Feel tired	
Tingling in my feet – brief the first day of chemo, went away	

Bring this list with you to your oncology appointment. If the person doing triage asks you if you've had any side effects, start by telling them about whatever symptoms are on your "Can't live with/Still ongoing list." That way, you make sure these issues are prioritized and your doctor will address them. After that, feel free to mention your "Can live with/ Improved on their own side effects," but make sure to mention that these side effects were *tolerable* or *improved on their own.* If you feel overwhelmed by doing this verbally, simply hand the triage person both lists. The triage person will ask you more questions about your symptoms and then communicate with your doctor.

How will this method of communicating help you? First, by prioritizing and highlighting your severe side effects, you help me know what to focus on—specifically, which symptoms are bothering you the most. At the same time, this method of communication allows you to still inform me about more minor side effects, so that as your cancer doctor, I'm still "in the loop." Having a structured way of reporting symptoms can be enormously helpful for your doctor to understand and treat your side effects.

MR. GEOFFREY'S STORY

Mr. Geoffrey was a 62-year-old man with stage 3 colon cancer. He was receiving chemotherapy every two weeks and sailing through treatment. Every time he came for an office visit, my nurse would tell me, "Mr. Geoffrey's doing well. He has some nausea for a couple of days after his treatment, but he takes his nausea meds and it's tolerable. Same with his constipation. He says it usually happens around the third day of his treatment, but he takes his stool softeners and it gets better."

One day, my nurse came in shaking her head. "What's wrong?" I asked.

"Mr. Geoffrey's mouth looks *awful*," she said. "He's got sores on his lips and the back of his throat. He says they popped up two days ago and look worse now.

He says he's not able to eat or drink and the pain is intolerable. He's lost about six pounds since his last visit."

"Poor guy," I said. "Mr. Geoffrey *never* complains. Let's go take a look."

Fifteen minutes later, I had diagnosed Mr. Geoffrey with an oral shingles outbreak. I sent a prescription to his pharmacy for an oral numbing medication as well as an anti-viral medication. I also suggested that he pick up L-Lysine, an oral supplement that could help prevent additional outbreaks. Otherwise, I advised him to keep doing what he was doing to manage his nausea and constipation.

Happy that we were doing something to treat his mouth pain, he thanked me and headed downstairs to receive his chemotherapy.

By describing his mouth pain as *ongoing* and *intolerable*, Mr. Geoffrey focused our attention on his most acute, concerning symptoms. Because of this, I did not waste our office visit discussing his nausea and constipation, both of which were present but *tolerable*. Instead, I spent our visit addressing the issue he was most concerned about. The end result? He was happy with the interaction, I was happy with the interaction, and above all, he got the medical care he required.

What if you want to discuss *all* your side effects? What if they *all* impact your quality of life?

Unfortunately, often time is limited. If you wish to discuss all your side effects with your doctor, you may end up frustrated if your doctor prioritizes some symptoms and ignores other symptoms. Second, the side effects that you experience directly impact my decisions regarding your chemotherapy. If you tell me that you have experienced 20 severe and disabling side effects from your treatment, I am probably going to stop your treatment or change your chemotherapy dose.

In medicine, everything is about the side effects, or risks, versus the benefits. You make risk versus benefit analyses in your head every day. You debate if buying that sweater that you saw is worth the price. You debate whether to eat at that restaurant you love, although you know it gives you heartburn. Whenever I consider chemotherapy for a patient, I weigh treatment side effects versus treatment benefits. If I feel the benefits outweigh the risks, I continue with treatment. If I feel that the risks outweigh the benefits, I stop chemotherapy or change the chemotherapy dose.

If you feel that you truly had 20 life-altering, intolerable side effects, then yes, absolutely, please tell me about them. I will do my best to address them and get you feeling better. However, the best way to fix 20 intolerable side effects is to remove the treatment that caused them in the first place—your chemotherapy. If there are many other treatment options available to you, changing your chemotherapy regimen may be easy and recommended. However, if chemotherapy options are limited, you may need to make a difficult decision. Are the side effects worth the treatment?

At the end of the day, continue to discuss your symptoms and side effects with your oncologist. Your oncologist cares about you and wants to make your life better. However, use the above technique to prioritize discussing your worst symptoms. By highlighting your most active issues, you will improve your communication with your doctor, and make sure that you are heard accurately and adequately.

Define Your Agenda

Aside from chemotherapy side effects, you may have important questions or topics you feel need to be addressed by your doctor at your appointment. How can you make sure these issues are discussed?

On most days, as your doctor, I walk into your appointment with a specific agenda in mind. I know that by the end of your visit, I need to review your labs, discuss new issues, and schedule your follow up appointment. In my mind, I allot a certain amount of time to each of these segments. As the clock continues to tick, if I find that we are running out of time, I will move on to my next discussion point.

As a patient, you may have a different agenda for your visit than your doctor. Because of this, you may feel that you are being rushed through your appointment, or that you have not had your questions addressed. If this is the case, there are a couple of things you can do to help the situation.

First, define your agenda. What is the most important topic you need to discuss at your appointment? Perhaps you had a question about your treatment or a particular concern about your chemotherapy. If you have two or three issues that you feel need to be discussed that is fine—but limit your list to no more than two or three items.

Second, briefly tell the nurse or medical assistant doing your visit triage the issues you wish to discuss. Often, the nurse and medical assistant is reporting directly to your doctor, so they will give your doctor a "heads up." That way, your doctor is prepared to address your questions or concerns.

Finally, remind your doctor at the beginning of the visit that you have specific questions you wish to discuss. This way, mentally, your doctor is "budgeting" the appropriate amount of time to answer each question. You can simply say, "I have a question I'd like to ask whenever you are ready." Your doctor will say, "Sure!" and either address your questions at that moment or a little later during your appointment. If you have two or three issues you wish to discuss, specifically tell your doctor, "I have two questions," or "I have three questions," so that way your doctor knows how many issues are on the table for discussion.

What if you have more than three questions? What if each question requires a very in-depth, long conversation? You have a couple of options at that point. If you have pages of questions, you will need to decide which ones are the most important to have addressed and narrow your questions down accordingly. Alternatively, you can call ahead and see if your doctor's office can adjust your appointment time to allot for more time with your doctor. For instance, your doctor's office may be able to change your appointment from a 15 minute time slot to a 30 minute appointment time slot. Sometimes this will not be an option due to high patient volumes, but you can certainly ask. You can also schedule a follow up appointment with your office's nurse practitioner. Often, nurse practitioners will have longer office visits than physicians and more flexible availability. Finally, you can try scheduling your appointment for the last visit of the day. If you are the last patient of the day, your doctor may be able to spend more time with you without inconveniencing other patients.

As your doctor, I want to make sure you feel heard and respected. I will try to sit down with you and answer your questions and address your concerns. Time is often limited, and sometimes I will not be able to spend as much time with you as you (and I!) would like. However, by following the above recommendations, you can make sure that your most pressing and important issues are addressed.

It is Okay to Switch Cancer Doctors

If you do not feel comfortable with your doctor, despite giving the relationship ample time to develop, it is okay to find a new doctor.

Sometimes, it comes down to communication style. You may feel like your doctor does not spend enough time with you, or does not answer your questions. Sometimes it boils down to feeling more comfortable with a female doctor, or vice versa. At the end of the day, your cancer doctor is trying to give you the best care possible. However, if you feel like you need to switch to another doctor, that's okay. As mentioned earlier, call your doctor's office and ask to speak to the office manager. Explain to the office manager why you are unhappy or uncomfortable with your current oncologist. The office manager will typically try to remedy the situation if possible. For instance, if your oncologist is always running late, the office manager may suggest scheduling your appointment as the first appointment of the day. However, if it's truly a matter that cannot be fixed with a simple solution, the office manager will assist with transitioning you to another oncologist within the practice.

While it may be disheartening to learn that one of my patients has elected to go to another doctor, I do not take it personally. I can usually tell when a patient does not like me, or a family member does not trust me. It makes life better for you *and* me if you find an oncologist with whom you feel comfortable. I would prefer you to be happy with another oncologist than stay with me and be miserable.

With that in mind, *tell* the office manager the issue you have with your current doctor, and be honest. If the issue is that you simply feel your doctor is too young and inexperienced, tell the office manager, so that he or she can place you with an older doctor. If you feel that your doctor has too thick of an accent, or talks too quickly, tell the office manager. He or she will place you with someone who has a clearer communication style. If you have breast cancer and would feel more comfortable with a female doctor, let the office manager know. By clarifying the source of your discomfort, the practice can match you with a doctor better suited to your situation.

Examples of Acceptable Reasons to Ask to Switch Doctors
You feel more comfortable with female/male providers
You are hard of hearing and have difficulty understanding your current provider
Your current provider does not spend enough time with you
Your current provider does not answer your questions
Your current provider does not explain things clearly

There are two important points to remember if you are thinking about switching doctors. First, as cancer doctors, we often have to give bad news. *No one* wants to hear bad news. I do not like giving bad news! But the truth has to be told. If the reason you want to switch doctors is because your oncologist gave you bad news, you may be trying to run from the truth. Switching to another doctor will not help the situation, and may actually delay your care. Remember that it is better to have a doctor that shares the truth with you, no matter how bluntly, than a doctor that does not communicate the truth at all.

Second, if you have switched oncologists more than three times, you might need to step back and evaluate your own behavior.

MS. KAREN'S STORY

Ms. Karen had a lot of issues. As a 77-year-old woman with stage 4 rectal cancer, she had been living with metastatic cancer for almost five years. Over the course of five years, she had already gone through three different oncologists within my practice. I happened to see her one day when her usual oncologist was on vacation. While examining her in the office, I made small talk, asking about her grandchildren and her vacation plans.

"I like you so much more than my other doctor," she said. "Can I switch to you?"

I told her to talk to our office manager, as our office policy is to allow patients to switch oncologists if necessary. She made the necessary phone calls, and within the next two weeks, I assumed her care.

At first, things were fine. She was responding well to treatment and was having minimal side effects.

After a couple of appointments, however, I noticed that things were changing. She was showing up later and later for her appointments. Instead of arriving early for her labs, she would arrive at the lab at the exact time her appointment with me was scheduled. Soon she was arriving **10, 20**, even 30 minutes late for her appointments.

She insisted on changing her dose and schedule for chemotherapy, even though I told her that I recommended against it. I would work with my secretary to adjust her schedule, and then a couple of days later she would call back and say that she changed her mind. Eventually, after she had changed her chemotherapy regimen from every other week to once every four weeks, her cancer markers rose. Panicking, she demanded repeat imaging with a PET/CT.

At this point, I decided that I had to intervene. Part of the issue here was my fault; I was letting her lead her care. It was easier to say "Yes," to her than to say "No." However, what she needed now was a doctor, not a friend. So I stepped in and stepped up.

Ms. Karen was *not* happy. She called our office on the hour, every hour, demanding to have a special type of scan known as a PET/CT ordered. I talked to her and explained that I did not recommend a PET/CT. A PET/CT would tell me the same thing her cancer markers were telling me—that her cancer had gotten worse. I recommended switching her therapy back to every other week because it had previously been working and she had been tolerating it well. If her cancer markers did not improve within a couple of weeks, I would be happy to order a PET/CT. If she did not wish to receive treatment as I recommended it—that was absolutely her choice. However, just like I could not *force* her to receive treatment, she could not *force* me to order her scans. I advised her that if she was unsatisfied with her care, she could talk to our office manager—and if she wished, she could change cancer doctors again.

Thus, I joined the long list of Ms. Karen's ex-oncologists.

Ms. Karen was a nice lady. She was actually doing incredibly well with her cancer. *But*...her erratic behavior and lack of insight into her disease made it difficult to care for her. Her own behavior was negatively impacting the quality of her care.

If you have had to switch oncologists more than three times, consider your past behavior. Consider what ways you might be hurting your own care. Remember, while I would love to be considered your friend, at the end of the day, I am your doctor first.

In summary, if you are dissatisfied with the care you have received, switching to another oncologist is easy and typically requires nothing more than a phone call. Be open and honest about the reasons you want to change doctors, so that you can be matched with a new doctor that will better match your needs. Remember that sometimes your doctor may tell you news that you do not want to hear. However, that is part of the job, and your oncologist will walk beside you through both the good times *and* the bad times.

℞ Continue to See Your Primary Care Doctor (PCP)

Between visits with your oncologist and chemotherapy, you most likely feel that you spend your entire life at the doctor's office. Do you really need to keep seeing your primary care doctor during this time?

The answer is: Yes! I'm sorry. I know that going to see yet another doctor is the last thing you want to do at this time. But in reality, I am a specialist—I focus on cancer care. Your cholesterol is the last thing on my mind when I am making decisions regarding your chemotherapy. That being said, *someone* has to pay attention to your cholesterol! Not to mention your diabetes, high blood pressure, glaucoma, etc.

Another important reason to continue seeing your PCP is for medication refills. Often, patients will ask me to refill medications for them while they are receiving chemotherapy. "Dr. DeRidder," I'll hear, "I've run out of my blood pressure medication. Can you refill it?" Or, "I've developed another yeast infection. Can you send me a prescription?" If the medication is one that I am familiar with, or the condition is one that I am comfortable treating, typically I have no problem with writing a prescription. However, if the medication is a controlled substance prescribed by another doctor, such as pain medications, or one that I am unfamiliar with, such as certain diabetes medications, the answer will be, "I'm sorry, I think you need to call your primary care doctor."

Sometimes patients will ask me about conditions that are not necessarily related to their cancer treatment. "Dr.

DeRidder," I'll hear, "You mentioned my kidney function is abnormal. What do I need to do about that?" Or, "I've noticed that my sugars have been running high on my labs. Do I need to start taking anything for that?" These issues, while important, are not always directly related to your cancer treatment. In these situations, I will always refer you back to your primary care doctor.

So please, yes, continue to see your primary care doctor so you can receive the best primary care possible.

Be Nice

As your cancer care team, we understand better than most what you are going through, and we are doing everything possible to help you thrive. With that in mind, there are a couple of small, simple ways that you can show your respect and appreciation for your cancer team.

1. *Be on time.* I know this might seem like a double standard. "Dr. DeRidder," you say, "my doctor is always running twenty minutes behind! Why can't I just arrive twenty minutes late to my appointment?"

However, there are a lot of hidden steps that go into your doctor being able to step foot into the exam room. The process of getting you checked in at the front desk, getting your labs drawn, and performing your vital signs can take up to an hour. If you show up 20 minutes late to your appointment, the whole process gets pushed back. A 20 minute late arrival can set your doctor's schedule back by an hour.

Being punctual for your appointments shows your doctor that you respect his or her time. In return, your doctor will do his or her best to respect yours.

2. *Be polite to support staff.* Yes, I know, they ask you a lot of strange and repetitive questions. It is easy to get frustrated having to repeat your medication list for the hundredth time or to feel insulted when someone asks you if you have any stress in your life (what a silly question to ask someone diagnosed with cancer, right?). However, this is part of our jobs, and we all play a role in your cancer care. Be kind to the people taking care of you during your darkest hour. Remember that kindness is contagious, and that even a small act of kindness can have an enormous impact.

3. *Say "Thank you."* Taking care of you is part of our job. However, our jobs are not easy. When you say, "Thank you," it acknowledges the sacrifices we make and the little ways we go above and beyond to take care of you. Knowing that you appreciate our time and care truly inspires us to continue our difficult field of medicine.

WHAT YOU HAVE LEARNED IN THIS SECTION

Summary:

- Learn the difference between complaining and reporting. Break down your side effects as "tolerable/

improved on their own" and "intolerable/ongoing." Use these classifications to help you better communicate your symptoms to your oncologist.

- If you have questions or concerns you wish to discuss with your oncologist, give your doctor a heads up at the beginning of your appointment. That way he or she can budget an appropriate amount of time to discuss your issues.
- If you feel like you and your doctor are not "clicking," it's okay to switch doctors.
- Keep seeing your primary care doctor for non-cancer-related health concerns.
- Take time to thank the team caring for you.

Over the past couple of pages, I have reviewed ways to communicate with your oncologist, including how to categorize your symptoms and side effects so that you can quickly convey information to your doctor, as well as how to "define your agenda" for your office visit. I have also discussed what to do if you find yourself unhappy with your oncology care. Finally, I have discussed ways you can show your cancer team that you appreciate their care.

In the next section, I will cover some of the emotional, mental, and financial side effects of chemotherapy. While it would be impossible to discuss all of the side effects of chemotherapy that fall into these categories, there are a couple of topics I believe applicable to every person diagnosed with cancer. I will highlight these topics in the following section.

Your Mental, Emotional and Financial Health

"So you think it'd be okay?" Ms. Elizabeth asked me.

"Well, I would probably avoid the manicure part, just given the fact that your immune system is slightly suppressed. Otherwise, I think the rest sounds completely fine." For the past three years, Ms. Elizabeth had taken her three daughters out for lunch and manicures the day before her eldest returned to college. She had come into clinic today asking if they would have to cancel their annual tradition.

"Oh, good," she said with relief. "I know it sounds silly, but...it really is such a special day for us. I knew that we probably couldn't do everything we usually do. I mean, usually, we go out shopping for a couple of hours in the morning, but I just don't have the energy for that right now. But I thought lunch would be fine. What if instead of a manicure I got a massage instead?"

"That'd be fine," I told her. "Just let them know that you have a port. Whoever is doing the massage should avoid manipulating the area where the port is."

"Well, maybe we'll just watch a movie at home or something instead," she said after some thought. "I could care less about the manicure part. The most important part for me is spending time with my girls."

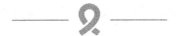

Adjusting to life with chemotherapy will take both time and patience. For many patients, making the adjustment from "life before chemotherapy" to "life during chemotherapy" can be an incredibly difficult transition. Some traditions, like Ms. Elizabeth's, will need to be modified, while others can occur as planned. Some old behaviors will have to change, while some new behaviors will need to be learned. However, the transition between "life before chemotherapy" and "life during chemotherapy" can be done, and eventually, even my most anxious and medically frail patients fall into a routine when it comes to their treatment. Once this transition is accomplished, many patients find that they are tougher and braver than they had ever believed.

The goal of this chapter is to introduce a couple of topics that I believe are important in making the transition from "pre-chemo" life to "life during chemo." It is important for me to again stress that this book is written from the perspective of a cancer doctor, not a cancer survivor. There are many books written by cancer survivors that will more intimately detail the emotional journey through cancer diagnosis and treatment. In this book, the issues I address are the questions I am most commonly asked in my clinic, and the answers I most commonly provide to my patients. The goal of this book is to provide you, as a patient, information that may not be available from other resources.

WHAT YOU WILL GET OUT OF THIS SECTION

Expect a new normal[12]	A reminder that you can do this (really, you can).
Fight for your life[13]	A reminder that the most important person in this fight is you.
Believe	A discussion about the role of faith during cancer treatment.
Financial toxicity	A brief discussion about an important side effect of cancer care.
Financial preparation	How to make sure your POA has access to your financial records.
Prescriptions and prior authorization	A word about the prior authorization process and some prescription resources.

---

[12] This section only applies to patients with early stage (stage 1, 2 and 3) cancers. If you have been diagnosed with stage 4 cancer, please turn to Chapter 7 for more information.

[13] This section only applies to patients with early stage (stage 1, 2 and 3) cancers. If you have been diagnosed with stage 4 cancer, please turn to Chapter 7 for more information.

Expect a New Normal

A few years ago, there was a commercial on television for a chemotherapy pill to treat breast cancer. In the commercial, the fictional patient says, "My life is different now. But this is my new normal."

After starting chemotherapy, within a few cycles, you should be able to predict side effects and establish a rhythm to your days. While your life might look different than it did pre-cancer diagnosis, you too should be able to establish a "new normal" (if you were diagnosed with stage 4 cancer, please refer to the chapter titled, "Stage 4 cancer" and the section "Finding a new normal with stage 4 cancer").

Your "new normal" may be very different than your life pre-cancer diagnosis. You will likely be unable to do some of the activities you used to enjoy. Chemotherapy is tough. However, these changes will hopefully be temporary. Realize that while your life may be more difficult than it was prior to chemotherapy, you are investing in your future. We are giving you treatment with the goal of preventing your cancer from coming back. If the side effects of your chemotherapy are manageable, in my mind, they are worth enduring in hopes of achieving a future that is cancer-free.

Learn the rhythm of your treatment. There will be days that you feel bad—and there will also be days that you feel fine. There will be times when you have to stay indoors— and there will be times when you can go out to dinner with friends and family. Your life will be dramatically different than it was before your cancer diagnosis. However, in some ways, often the most important ways, it will remain the same. You will learn to manage your side effects. You will learn to take your nausea medication around the clock on certain days of your cycle. You will learn to take certain days easy, and to plan events for days you know you will feel fine. Ultimately, you and your doctor will find what works best to keep you healthy.

Remember that this is all temporary. You will adjust, and you will rise to the situation. This will be your new normal— for now.

Fight for Your Life

If your cancer is potentially curable, I will do everything I can to get you safely through your chemotherapy and into remission. However, I can only do so much. I am an external factor in your cancer success story. The most important person in this story is *you*. I will help you fight, but I cannot fight for you.

I know that I am not walking in your shoes. I know that I am not the one who has to deal with new side effects. I know that you are tired, lonely, and scared.

However, I also know that the patients who fight are the patients who live.

As a cancer doctor, I have treated many, many patients, and I have seen the difference between those who try and *keep trying*—and those who do not. There will be times when you do not want to eat. There will be times when you do not want to get out of bed. You must force yourself to eat. To walk. To get out of bed. You must find the inner will to push through your symptoms and maintain your performance status. Of course, I will try to do what I can to relieve your chemotherapy side effects. However, there is no pill that I can give you that will make you feel 100 percent normal. There is no medication in the world I can give you to replace your own motivation.

▼

MR. THOMAS'S STORY

Mr. Thomas was a 67-year-old man with stage 4 colon cancer. Though he had stage 4 disease, he only had one area of cancer in his liver, and there was still a potential chance of cure. At our initial consultation appointment, Mr. Thomas was determined to cure his cancer.

"Let's do whatever we need to do to kick this thing's butt," he exclaimed.

I started him on neoadjuvant chemotherapy to shrink his cancer. Chemotherapy was fairly bumpy, but we managed to get the kinks worked out. He made it through four cycles of treatment. When I repeated his scans, we found that his cancer had shrunk by over 50 percent. I referred him to a surgeon for evaluation, and the surgeon agreed that he was a good candidate for partial liver resection. He would need chemotherapy afterward to try to kill any residual cancer cells, but there was still a chance that he could be cured.

"This is going to be a major surgery," I reminded him. "They are removing part of your liver. The liver will grow back slowly, but there is also a chance that this could throw your body into liver failure. You could get a bad infection, or you could even die during the surgery. However, by removing the part of your liver with the cancer in it, there is about a forty percent chance that you will remain cancer-free at five years."

"Let's do it," Mr. Thomas agreed.

Initially, he did well with his surgery. Unfortunately, after surgery his recovery was plagued by complications. His liver did not heal, and he developed something called a biloma, a collection of bile in the liver that does not drain properly. He required placement of a chronic drain running from the liver to the outside of his body. His wife had to empty the drain bags daily, or the bile would back up. Multiple times, his surgeon rescanned him in hopes that the biloma had resolved, only to find it still present. Mr. Thomas had pain from the drain, as well as nausea. During this time, his surgeon and primary care doctor managed his symptoms.

Approximately two months later, Mr. Thomas showed back up in my office, finally ready to resume chemotherapy. "I'm finally drain free, doc," he said happily.

"You know," he elaborated, "I kept going back to my primary care doctor. Every other week I was in his office, telling him, 'I'm so tired,' or, 'I don't want to eat, food doesn't taste good.' Eventually, my doc said, 'Thomas—you need to learn to live with these issues or be referred to hospice. Because there is nothing else I can do.'"

Mr. Thomas smiled at me. "I want to live. So I'm doing my best to eat even though food doesn't taste great. I'm trying to stay active, even though I'm more tired than I used to be. Every day I try to walk farther around the block with my wife. When I went back to my surgeon, my last scan looked better, and he was able to remove the drain."

I nodded in understanding. Almost every patient walks in the door saying "I want to fight." However, as the side effects stack up, the will to fight can wane. Patients can get stuck in a chemotherapy limbo, where they are too scared to stop but too weak to keep going. If a cancer is incurable, stopping chemotherapy at that point is very appropriate. However, if a cancer is potentially curable, at that point the patient needs to make a choice.

Fight for your life, or let it go.

Mr. Thomas chose to fight. Cancer, chemotherapy, and surgery had knocked him down, but he decided that he would drag himself off the floor and stand back up again. It wasn't easy, it wasn't pleasant, and it wasn't fast. While his surgeon and primary care doctor did what they could to help him, in the end, he had to figure out a way to mentally, emotionally, and physically cope with his side effects. And he did.

I really admired Mr. Thomas's determination. I also really admired Mr. Thomas's primary care doctor for being honest and upfront with him. The truth was harsh, but it was what Mr. Thomas needed to hear. I truly believe that by having this discussion with him, Mr. Thomas's primary care doctor saved his life.

At the end of the day, modern medicine has its limits. There is no pill I can give you that will make you feel totally normal. There will be days that you feel bad—and there will be days that you feel good. There will be days that you feel like you can conquer mountains and days that you feel like giving up. I wish that I could make you feel better, and I will do everything I can to alleviate your symptoms. Ultimately, however, there will be side effects, and the only person that can get you through your therapy is you. Earlier in this chapter, I mentioned that you will develop a "new normal." This is your life—for now. You must find a way to cope with your new normal.

What if you cannot find a new normal? What if *nothing* is worth the symptoms that you are currently experiencing? At that point, you will have to make a difficult choice. Keep going with chemotherapy—or stop, knowing the potential risks. If you can accept that we may be sacrificing efficacy for tolerability, we can certainly change or even stop your therapy. However, if you expect to be cured of your cancer, you may need to temporarily sacrifice some quality of life for the ultimate goal of being cancer free.

Believe

One powerful thing that can help you during this time is faith. Believe in God. Believe in Allah. Believe in Jesus, believe in Krishna, the Goddess, Thor, believe in the healing color of purple. Believe in whatever you want, as long as you believe in something.

Cancer is a game-changer. Your life changes in a moment and things will never be the same again. I cannot tell you how many times I have heard a patient say, "I can't believe this is happening to me. I just...*insert blank*." Retired, got married, graduated from college, had a baby. Unfortunately, I have heard it all. Cancer is stubborn, impatient, and it does not compromise.

Believing in a higher power can help mitigate the feeling of helplessness that can occur with a cancer diagnosis. Believing that there is a plan for everything and that everything happens for a reason, even if we cannot understand that reason, can help you regain your sense of control and purpose in life. I strongly believe that patients who have faith in a higher power live healthier and happier lives. However, while it is important to believe in a higher power, it is also important to be realistic.

MS. LILLIE'S STORY

Ms. Lillie was a 77-year-old lifelong smoker with stage 4 lung cancer. She was a devout Christian, and from the very beginning told me, "It's in God's hands, sweetie." That being said, Ms. Lillie had a lot to live for and wanted to be aggressive with her treatment. She had a good performance status and was a candidate for chemotherapy, with the understanding that chemotherapy could not cure her disease, only slow it down. We treated her with both chemotherapy and immunotherapy, with initially good results. However, as the months went by, her performance status decreased due to both her cancer and the side effects of her treatment. Throughout this, she was hopeful and cheerful, to the point that I took care to remind her periodically that I could not cure her. I told her that I did not want her to be blindsided, but that at some point I would not be able to offer her further treatment. She accepted this gracefully, but always countered back, "I'm still hoping for a miracle."

One day, her family brought her to my office in a wheelchair. She was no longer able to get around more than a couple of feet without wearing oxygen. On reviewing her vital signs, I noticed that she had continued to lose weight. "Food just doesn't have a taste anymore," she told me. Her most recent scan had shown that her cancer was growing again, and had spread to several additional areas.

She looked at me and said, "Dr. DeRidder, I just don't know what's going on. Everything seems like it's falling apart." I looked at her scan and then looked at her. I did not have any comforting words for her. She was right. She was no longer a candidate for any chemotherapy, and her cancer was progressing rapidly.

Eventually, I said to her quietly, "Ms. Lillie...I think you're dying."

She was quiet for a moment, and then nodded her head. "That's what I thought." She smiled sadly. "You know, I haven't given up that God may grant me a miracle. But...the miracle may have been that I lived a long, wonderful life. Either way, I think I've been pretty blessed."

Shortly thereafter, Ms. Lillie enrolled in home hospice. She lived for another month, and then passed away peacefully surrounded by her family.

The purpose of this story is not to be sad or to take away hope. The purpose of this story is to remind you that faith does not come with guarantees. The outcome you hope for may not be the outcome God has planned for you. We all—including myself—hope for a miracle when it comes to healing cancer. However, at the end of the day, the miracle may not be the life you gain, but the life you have already lived.

Believe in something higher than yourself. Prepare for the worst, but hope and pray for the best. Believe that God has a plan for you and that no matter where this road goes, the destination will be all right.

Financial Toxicity

Unfortunately, **financial toxicity** is a side effect of cancer care that often gets forgotten. Financial toxicity refers to the cumulative cost of cancer treatment and includes co-pays, cost of medications, and hospital bills. As a doctor, I do not often directly deal with the financial underbelly of cancer care. However, most patients do have to pay a significant price to receive necessary treatment.

What can you do to reduce your financial toxicity? The first place to start is by asking for help. Ask your cancer doctor if you can speak to a social worker or case manager. Often, the case manager working with your doctor will have access to small gift cards to gas stations, grocery stores, and local franchises. These can help alleviate a bit of your day-to-day expenses. If transportation to and from your treatment is an issue for you, your social worker or case manager can also help you apply for medical transport. You may also qualify for free access to a gym, free mastectomy bras, and free wigs depending on your cancer stage and diagnosis.

In my hospital, depending on your income, you also may potentially qualify for hospital financial assistance. For individuals who make below a certain income, my hospital will actually cover some of your cancer related hospital bills. The financial department at your oncologist's office can also help you apply for Medicare and Medicaid.

If you were working at the time of your cancer diagnosis, it is very likely that you will need to take some time off from work during your cancer treatment. This leave of absence may be temporary, or it may be more permanent. Regardless, there will *always* be paperwork necessary to obtain a leave of absence. Please, go to your human resource department and inquire about the paperwork necessary to apply for a leave of absence. Bring the paperwork back to your oncologist, and your oncologist will be happy to fill out the forms. Please be aware that we typically require a one to two-week turnaround for completing work-related documents.

If you are taking a leave of absence from work, you may also need to apply for **disability benefits**. Applying for disability benefits is typically done through your social services department. You can visit www.ssa.gov for more information.

If your oncologist prescribed an oral form of chemotherapy, there is a chance that your cancer team can apply for financial assistance from the drug's pharmaceutical company. You will have to submit your financial information and prior tax information, but you may qualify for either free drug or heavily discounted medication.

If you are a veteran, you should also consider enrolling for benefits at your closest Veteran's Administration (VA) hospital. As a veteran, you will likely qualify for care at your local VA oncology clinic, where your care might actually be free. If you are located more than a certain distance from your closest VA oncology clinic, the VA may actually pay for you to be treated locally at a non-VA oncology clinic.

Sometimes, patients feel uncomfortable discussing financial issues with their medical team. Don't be! As a doctor, I am comfortable dealing with all aspects of a patient's care. If you are struggling with the financial aspect of treatment, please let me know. I cannot and will not spend your entire appointment discussing money matters. However, if I am at least aware of the problem, I will help in any way that I can. Bottom line, while your treatment may still cost you some money, there are many financial resources available. *Your bottom line may be less than you think.*

Financial Preparation

At some point during your cancer treatment, you may need to be hospitalized for a short period of time. It may be a planned admission, or it may be an emergent admission. Regardless, the last thing you need to worry about during that time is missed bill payments.

With this in mind, if you have been diagnosed with cancer, I recommend you write down your username and password to major accounts, including your utilities, bank accounts, student loans, and car payments. Give your power of attorney (POA) a copy of your online account usernames and passwords, and a list of your monthly expected bill payments. Include with this information a copy of your will and the legal paperwork identifying them your POA. Write

"Financial Documents" on the front, and tell your POA to keep this file someplace safe but easily accessible. This way, if life takes an unexpected turn, you can rest easy knowing that someone you trust has access to your accounts and can handle your affairs if you are unavailable. Obviously, this has to be someone you trust completely with your finances. Typically, this person is your designated POA.

Common Accounts Your POA Should Have Access To in an Emergency:
Bank accounts (i.e. Bank of America, Capital One, Wells Fargo, etc.)
Loan accounts (i.e. student loans, personal loans, business loans, mortgages, etc.)
Email account
Utilities (electric, water, etc.)

Common Recurring Payments:
Mortgage/rent
Car payments
Other loans (i.e, student loans, personal loans, business loans, etc.)
Childcare (i.e., daycare payments, nanny, school tuition, etc.)
Insurance payment (Health, dental, care, homeowners, etc.)
Utilities (electric, water, etc.)

MS. CASSANDRA'S STORY

Ms. Cassandra was a 73-year-old woman with stage 4 breast cancer. She was receiving chemotherapy and doing well. One winter day she showed up at my office with bronchitis. I prescribed her an oral antibiotic, hoping that I could treat her bronchitis before it turned into pneumonia. However, when she came back to clinic the following week, she had a low-grade fever, her cough was worse, and her oxygen levels were below normal. Based on her low-grade fever and symptoms, I recommended admitting her to the hospital.

Upon hearing my recommendation, Ms. Cassandra became very upset. "I can't be admitted to the hospital right now," she said. "Can I go home first and come back in a couple of hours?"

"Well, yes," I said, "but I wouldn't recommend it. Your heart rate is up and your oxygen levels are low. While at home, you could pass out, or get sicker. Also, by the time you come back, the clinic will be closed. You will have to go through the emergency room, and you might have to wait several hours in the emergency room before being admitted to a hospital room. As it is now, I have a hospital room waiting for you."

"It's just that the bills are due the first of the month," she said, "and Joe has no idea how to pay them." Joe, her husband, rarely accompanied her to her cancer appointments. He had several health issues of his own, and Ms. Cassandra tended to manage the financial aspects of their lives.

"Could Joe bring them to you while you are in the hospital?" I asked.

"I guess he could try," she said. "I'm not sure if he even knows where I keep the bills."

After going back and forth like this for a couple of minutes, she finally decided to leave against my medical advice so that she could go home and pay the bills. She returned to the emergency room several hours later, and in the early hours of the morning, was finally admitted to the hospital for treatment of her pneumonia.

If you manage your finances by paper instead of online, write down a list of all your recurring bills and your bank account numbers. Keep copies of major account statements as well as a copy of your will and legal paperwork identifying your POA. Write "Financial Documents" on the front, and either give it to your POA or place it in a safe, secure area where your POA can easily find it. Again, this has to be someone you trust completely with your finances.

Some people might think that this level of cautiousness is excessive, or even morbid. However, creating a financial "emergency file" for your POA is not at all morbid or bad luck. It's simply good planning! Of course, I hope that your life goes smoothly. However, my motto has always been "Prepare for the worst, and hope and pray for the best."

Prescriptions and Prior Authorization

If you go to your pharmacy to pick up a prescription and find out that the medication co-pay is astronomically high, most likely your insurance company requires something known as "**prior authorization**." Prior authorization is a process that insurance companies use to encourage doctors to prescribe only certain medications.

Many insurance companies have multiple medication co-pay tiers. Within these co-pay tiers, some medications are covered almost completely, while other medications are covered less so. Some medications may have an on-formulary alternative, meaning that your insurance company prefers that I order a specific medication as opposed to another. If your insurance company prefers that I prescribe their on-formulary alternative, they will make me obtain "prior authorization" for the non-formulary drug. In short, "prior authorization" is a process in which I have to justify to your insurance company why I need a particular medication as opposed to another.

Oncologists tend to be very aggressive in our attempts to obtain prior authorization. The reason for this is simple. Most of our treatments are life or death in nature. If I am prescribing a certain medication, it is typically because that medication is the best drug for the condition I am treating. However, I have had many patients where the insurance company has ultimately not covered the medication, no matter how passionately or logically I have argued.

If you go to your pharmacy and you are told that your medication co-pay is much higher than normal, likely your insurance company wants prior authorization for that particular drug. Please do not assume that your doctor's office will be aware of the situation. Call your doctor's office, and let them know that your co-pay is too high and you cannot pick up the medication. Ask your doctor's office to find out if you need prior authorization for the medication, and to call you back. If it turns out that no prior authorization is necessary, and unfortunately you just have a high co-pay, ask your doctor's office if an alternative medication can be prescribed.

DR. DERIDDER'S STORY

Approximately a year ago, my doctor wrote me a prescription for a week of antibiotics. When I went to the pharmacy, the pharmacy told me that the cost for 14 pills would be 100 dollars. My insurance company was refusing to pay for the antibiotics.

With that news, I went to the website GoodRx. GoodRx is a free to use website that tracks prescription drug prices and offers medication coupons. Nearly every pharmacy in the U.S. participates with GoodRx. If you search the GoodRx website for your medication, you will see the cost of your medication at several of your local pharmacies.

Using GoodRx, I looked up how much the antibiotic would cost at pharmacies in my local area. Amazingly, 14 pills of the antibiotic at my local grocery pharmacy would only cost $14.50. I called my doctor's office and asked them to resend the prescription to the grocery pharmacy. I went to the pharmacy and presented my GoodRx coupon on my phone. I paid $14.50, went home with my 14 pills of antibiotics, and got better.

While GoodRx cannot solve everyone's prescription medication problems, it can certainly help in some situations.[14] Give it a try. You might be amazed at the difference between what you are *currently* paying and what you *could* be paying.

Finally, if you are a veteran, please enroll for benefits at your local VA hospital. Often, veterans qualify for discounted medications, and this is a benefit that can save you hundreds, if not thousands, of dollars. Of note, the VA pharmacy does require that any prescription filled at a VA pharmacy be written by a VA physician. Therefore, you will also need to sign up for a VA primary care doctor. Typically, I will write a script for a medication, fax the prescription to your VA primary care doctor, and your VA primary care

---

[14] GoodRx cannot be combined with your health insurance or programs like Medicare or Medicaid. I do not own any financial stock in GoodRx and receive no compensation for promoting its services.

doctor will then send another script to the VA pharmacy. The medication will then be available for you to pick up, or sent to you through the mail.

WHAT YOU HAVE LEARNED IN THIS SECTION

Summary:

- You will develop a new pattern and flow for your daily routine. Remember that this is all temporary. You will adjust, and you will rise to the occasion. This will be your new normal—for now.
- Stay motivated.
- Believe in a higher power or something bigger than yourself.
- Talk to your doctor if you are struggling financially.
- Designate a power of attorney (POA).

In this section, I have discussed some of the mental, emotional, and financial issues that can affect your life during your chemotherapy. Hopefully, some of the points discussed in this chapter will make your life easier as your transition from "pre-chemo" life to "life during chemo."

In this next section, I will discuss some of the issues that can affect your physical health during chemotherapy.

Your Physical Health

"Our talk last week got me thinking more about massage," Ms. Elizabeth said. She was returning to clinic today for her sixth dose of her weekly chemotherapy. "My youngest daughter is really into yoga, and she keeps telling me that I should do it with her. I don't think I'm quite up for that, but I thought maybe something more relaxing, like a massage, would be nice."

"Sure," I said. "Like I mentioned last week, let them know that you're on cancer treatment and have a port. But other than that, there's no reason you can't get a massage. In fact, it will probably help with some of your fatigue."

"Though maybe I should do something like yoga," she laughed ruefully. "I always thought I would lose weight with chemo, but instead I've gained five pounds!"

I smiled at her. "That's not a bad thing. A little weight gain tells me that you are eating, which is good. I'd be much more worried if you were losing weight."

"Really?" she asked, looking surprised. "My primary doctor has always wanted me to lose ten pounds for my blood pressure."

"Yup," I told her, "I usually tell my patients to try to maintain their weight as much as possible. Now, I don't mind if you lose weight from exercise, or from changing your diet. However, most people lose weight during chemo from not eating. When that happens, you're not losing fat—you're losing muscle. And when you lose muscle, that's when you start getting weak."

"Oh, interesting," Ms. Elizabeth said. She laughed again. "Well, that's probably the first time a doctor has ever told me not to lose weight!"

Traditional chemotherapy works by putting stress on your body. These chemicals stress both cancer cells and healthy cells. Cancer cells are more fragile than healthy cells, so the hope is that ultimately, the cancer cells die, and your normal, healthy cells grow back.

There are small but vital ways you can assist your body with its recuperation and restoration process. In this chapter, I will discuss the role diet, weight, and hydration play in helping you thrive during your chemotherapy. I will also discuss the more controversial topics of supplements and complementary medicine, and the role they can have in your cancer care. Like I mentioned in my conversation with

Ms. Elizabeth, often complementary medicine can be safe and beneficial to your overall well-being. Of course, it's important to discuss any changes in your diet or exercise routine with your oncologist. That being said, with your doctor's support, I encourage you in finding new ways to nourish your body's recovery from chemotherapy.

WHAT YOU WILL GET OUT OF THIS SECTION

Diet recommendations	The concept of "calories over content," and what to eat if that concept does not apply to you.
Weight management	The importance of maintaining your weight during chemotherapy.
Hydrate	The role of hydration in maintaining your health.
Wash your hands	The importance of hand hygiene.
The role of supplements	The role of supplements in your cancer care.
The role of complementary medicine	The role of complementary medicine in your cancer care.

Diet Recommendations

"Is there anything special I should be eating while I'm receiving chemotherapy?"

As a cancer doctor, it is one of the questions I get asked most often by patients and their families. The answer is no...and yes.

Imagine this scenario. Mrs. Janice is a 70-year-old woman who comes into the office with her daughter and granddaughter. She was recently diagnosed with stage 3 lung cancer, and we are talking about initiating chemotherapy.

"Well," her 23-year-old vegan granddaughter says, "what changes in her diet can she make to help her fight cancer?"

At this point, I look at her grandmother, who currently weighs 100lbs. According to my records, she has already lost 20lbs over the past six months.

"I recommend she eat whatever she wants," I reply.

Well-meaning granddaughter looks frustrated. "What I mean," she says, "is that I've been a vegan for three years, so I'm pretty familiar with using diet to impact your health. Since my grandma was diagnosed with cancer, I've been reading a lot of information online. I know that some foods are high in antioxidants. I want to make sure she's on a diet to help boost her immune system."

This is usually where I introduce the concept of "calories over content." More important than the *type* of calories you are getting is making sure you are getting *enough* calories.

Think of it this way. Imagine you are recovering from the stomach flu. For the first time in days, you feel like you could keep some food down. In this moment, the food you crave the most is...kale? No. You want chicken noodle soup, toast, and mac and cheese. Your body is in need of comfort, so in turn, you reach for comfort food.

While receiving chemotherapy, it is very likely that your appetite will not be normal. You might find yourself eating half of your lunch instead of all it. You might start skipping snacks, skipping dessert, or skipping breakfast. Of course, when you eat less, you lose weight. Unfortunately, when you lose weight, you lose muscle, which in turn makes it harder for you to do your "activities of daily living." One of the most important factors influencing your treatment is your *performance status*. If you do not eat, you lose weight, and your performance status goes down. So at the end of the day, what do I want you to do? Eat!

"Dr. DeRidder," you say, "that doesn't answer my question. What *exactly* should I be eating?"

Whatever you feel like eating! If you sit down for dinner and the only thing you feel like eating is mashed potatoes, go for it. I would rather you eat 100 percent of a plate of mashed potatoes then only 25 percent of a salad, even if the salad does have more nutrients. If your performance status is on the line, I prefer calories over content.

So, sitting in the room with my 70-year-old patient and her family, I would recommend she focus on consuming calories to prevent further weight loss. If she keeps losing weight, she is going to become frailer, and at some point, she will no longer be a candidate for chemotherapy. I would prefer she focus on gaining weight rather than trying to reach some theoretical nutrient level.

If you need guidance on how to increase your caloric intake, ask your oncologist to refer you to a nutritionist or dietician. You can also search online for "high caloric diet for cancer patients." You will find a number of websites with helpful tips on increasing your caloric intake.

What if you are eating well and having no issues with maintaining your weight? What if you have finished your chemotherapy and are looking to improve your overall health?

Here is where the "...yes," portion of my original answer comes in. If you are *truly* getting in enough calories and your performance status is excellent, then...yes, there are certain foods I would recommend incorporating into your diet, and certain foods that I would recommend you avoid.

First, I would recommend foods high in protein, provided that your kidneys work normally. Protein is the building block for muscle, and we know that muscle = performance status.

Second, choose foods high in antioxidants. Antioxidants are substances that can protect your cells against free radicals. Free radicals are molecules that can cause DNA damage, which in turn can result in impaired healing and can even eventually lead to cancer. By eating a diet high in antioxidants, you will give your immune system a boost in fighting cancer.

Examples of Some Foods High in Antioxidants
Oatmeal
Blueberries, strawberries, raspberries, pomegranate juice, Asian pears
Pecans
Kale, spinach, purple cabbage, beets
Dark chocolate
Pinto beans

Finally, try to reduce your sugar intake. All cells in your body use sugar as fuel. However, cancer cells use a *significantly* higher amount of sugar compared to normal, healthy cells. By eating a diet heavy in sugar, you are feeding your body, but you are also feeding the cancer. Remember, though, if you are receiving chemotherapy, a diet low in sugar is *only* recommended if you are maintaining your weight and performance status.

Occasionally, some medications that we use for cancer treatment can actually *cause* weight gain. Patients receiving medications known as "**endocrine therapy**" may actually find that they are slowly gaining weight despite maintaining a normal diet. Endocrine therapy typically involves medications that change hormone levels to affect cancer cells. A side effect of endocrine therapy can be decreased metabolism, which in turn will cause weight gain. Patients receiving endocrine therapy often *will* have to watch their diet. One popular diet I recommend for patients receiving endocrine therapy, or for those who have completed che-motherapy, is **the Pink Ribbon Diet**.

The Pink Ribbon Diet is a lifestyle regimen created by Dr. Mary Flynn, a research dietitian and assistant professor at Brown Medical School. The Pink Ribbon Diet emphasizes a plant-based, olive-oil diet that can help manage weight gain, enable better control over blood sugar and cholesterol, and improve blood pressure. Recipes following the Pink Ribbon Diet can be found online, or you can buy *The Pink Ribbon Diet: A Revolutionary New Weight Loss Plan to Lower Your Breast Cancer Risk* on Amazon.

In addition to the Pink Ribbon Diet, there are a number of diet plans out there that promote themselves as hav-ing "anti-cancer properties." If you are maintaining your weight and performance status and want to try one of these "anti-cancer" diets, that is typically fine. Of course, every patient is different, and I would recommend you discuss your diet changes with your oncologist. Keep in mind that these alternative diets will likely cost extra money, time, and effort, and there may be little to no data to support these diets. However, it makes sense that diets high in vegetables and fruits are good for you, and may provide additional benefits when battling cancer.

In summary, if you have lost a significant amount of weight before starting chemotherapy, or you are having trouble maintaining your weight during chemotherapy, I prefer calories over content. Whatever you find appetizing, eat it!

Weight loss = muscle loss = loss of performance status. Maintaining your performance status is key to doing well with chemotherapy. That being said, if you are feeling well and your weight is stable, I would recommend steering towards a high protein, high anti-oxidant, and low sugar diet. Finally, if you are having trouble with weight gain because of your cancer treatment, or have already completed your cancer treatment, I would recommend the Pink Ribbon Diet or a diet that is high in fruits, vegetables, and lean proteins.

Weight Management

By now, you are probably familiar with the typical doctor's office routine. You go to the doctor's office and step on the scale. The doctor looks at the scale, looks at you, and says, "Hmm. You need to lose some weight."

Guess what? If you are receiving chemotherapy, *please stop losing weight.*

As previously mentioned, most patients receiving chemotherapy will have a diminished appetite. Unfortunately, while the medical field has developed many effective anti-nausea medications, our arsenal of appetite stimulants has not developed quite as robustly. In my experience, the appetite stimulants we prescribe work about half of the time. Because of this, it is very common that people lose weight during chemotherapy.

Finally, you think. One good side effect of chemotherapy! Time to dig my skinny pants out of the closet.

Not so fast! You see, chemotherapy changes your metabolism. So when you lose weight while receiving chemotherapy, it's not like losing weight from going to the gym, or from changing your diet. You're not losing fat. You're losing muscle. Losing muscle is dangerous because as you start losing muscle, you start saying things like, "I'm just more tired than I used to be." Or, "I don't have the energy I used to have." Normal activities, like going to the mailbox, suddenly make you winded. You find yourself taking more naps throughout the day.

Remember that discussion about performance status in Chapter 1? In short, weight loss tends to cause muscle loss, and muscle loss causes your performance status to go down. Unfortunately, as your performance status goes down, my ability to continue your chemotherapy disappears as well.

With that in mind, one of the most important things you can do for yourself is to remind yourself to eat. When you sit down for dinner, you may fill up quickly. Your sense of taste may be off. You might feel inclined to say, "I'm not hungry anymore. I'm not going to force myself." Or maybe, "Food just doesn't taste the same anymore."

However, you are fighting against a powerful adversary, and you need all the resources you can get. So force yourself to eat just a *couple* more bites. Do not make yourself sick or nauseous. Just make a conscious effort to eat a little more. Remind yourself in between meals that even if you do not *feel* like eating, you *have* to eat.

Of course, there are always exceptions to this rule. One exception is for patients on hospice, or on end of life care. Another exception is for patients who have finished chemotherapy and are in remission. If you have finished chemotherapy, you will likely notice gradual improvements in your appetite and taste. You will also notice your weight slowly increasing. If you lost a significant amount of weight before or during chemotherapy, this weight gain can be a good thing. However, it is possible to have "too much of a good thing." Excess weight can cause issues with high blood pressure, diabetes, and high cholesterol. You just fought to be cancer free. Let's make sure the rest of your body is in tip-top shape as well!

Similar concerns apply to patients who are receiving endocrine therapy. As previously mentioned, endocrine therapy typically involves medications that change hormone levels to affect cancer cells. A side effect of endocrine therapy can be decreased metabolism, which in turn will cause weight gain. This is concerning because weight gain has actually been linked to an increased risk of developing and dying from several types of cancer.[15]

If you have finished chemotherapy, or if you are currently receiving endocrine therapy, I would recommend the Pink Ribbon Diet. As mentioned previously, the Pink Ribbon Diet a lifestyle regimen created by Dr. Mary Flynn, a research dietitian and assistant professor at Brown Medical School. It

---

[15] Jiralerspong S, Goodwin PJ. Obesity and Breast Cancer Prognosis: Evidence, Challenges, and Opportunities. J Clin Oncol. 2016 Dec 10;34(35):4203-4216. doi: 10.1200/JCO.2016.68.4480.

emphasizes a plant-based, olive-oil diet that can help manage weight gain, enable better control over blood sugar and cholesterol, and improve blood pressure. Recipes following the Pink Ribbon Diet can be found online, or you can buy *The Pink Ribbon Diet: A Revolutionary New Weight Loss Plan to Lower Your Breast Cancer Risk* on Amazon.

In summary, I recommend against weight loss during chemotherapy. I understand the drive to improve your health during this time. However, your body is undergoing a tremendous amount of stress during chemotherapy. Rather than jeopardize your performance status, I would recommend holding off on weight loss until after you complete your treatment. After you complete chemotherapy, I encourage and applaud your weight loss efforts. If you are on endocrine therapy, I also encourage weight loss and recommend The Pink Ribbon Diet as a diet that can assist you in your health endeavors.

Hydrate

It's true. You need to drink more water.

Chemotherapy = chemicals. These chemicals have a purpose, to kill cancer cells. However, your body has to eventually get rid of these chemicals, as well as all the toxins released when cancer cells die. Your intestines, liver, and kidneys work as filters for your body. These organs typically neutralize and remove all the toxins floating around in your blood system that could potentially harm you. Guess how they do that? Through water! So when you get a hefty dose of chemotherapy, your liver, kidneys, and intestines are working overtime. Help them out. Drink more water.

How much water do you need to drink? The recommendation you have probably heard all your life is to drink eight glasses of eight ounces of water a day. If you are already drinking that much water, that's amazing! For the rest of you...you are not alone. Almost everyone is dehydrated. However, most people do not have the added stress of chemotherapy on their bodies. With the added stress of cancer treatment, a chronic state of dehydration can rapidly spiral into severe dehydration.

What does dehydration feel like? Queasiness, headaches, body aches, fatigue, and loss of appetite. Unfortunately, these symptoms are the same symptoms you can get from chemotherapy. In fact, many of the side effects people experience from chemotherapy are actually caused by dehydration.

One way you can encourage yourself to drink more water is to carry around a small, 8 ounce bottle of water. People often think that getting a large, liter size jug will help them hydrate more. Actually, this can backfire. Looking at the jug, you think, *There's no way I can finish this.* However, with a small, 8 ounce bottle of water, you finish the bottle and think, *I did it. One bottle down!* Then you go, fill it back up, and repeat. Do this eight times, and you have met your water quota for the day.

Another method to improve your hydration is to receive IV hydration throughout your chemotherapy cycle. I frequently schedule IV hydration for patients after chemotherapy.

MS. BARBARA'S STORY

Ms. Barbara was a 69-year-old woman receiving chemotherapy for stage 3 endometrial cancer. She typically received chemotherapy every three weeks on a Monday. The week of chemotherapy, she would return to clinic on Thursday and Friday for IV hydration. It meant more time spent at the oncology clinic for her, but receiving the sessions of IV hydration helped minimize nausea and fatigue after her treatments. The better she felt, the fewer delays in her treatment, and the easier it was for her to continue on with her normal, non-chemotherapy life.

If you have been struggling with symptoms of dehydration after receiving chemotherapy, ask your oncologist if it would be possible to schedule you for IV hydration a day or two after your treatment. You might be amazed at the difference a little extra fluid can make.

Wash Your Hands

While you are receiving chemotherapy, you will be more vulnerable to germs. These germs—bacteria, viruses, and mold—enter your body through your eyes, nose, and mouth. The most common vehicle germs use to gain access to your eyes, nose, and mouth is your hands. Washing your hands is one of the easiest and most effective ways to prevent getting sick. Wash your hands before eating, before touching your mouth, before picking your nose, and before rubbing your eyes.

"Dr. DeRidder! No one around me is sick," you protest. "I'll be fine."

While *you* may not be directly touching sick people all day, I guarantee you that sick people are touching the items that you touch. Imagine that a man with a cold sneezes into his hands, and then opens the door to a restaurant. A minute later, you open the restaurant door. After sitting down to eat, the waiter brings you some bread and dip. "Great," you say. "Let's dig in." You grab a roll and start eating. And as easily as that, the germs have gone from the man to the door, to your hands, and finally, to the inside of your body.

Sometimes, it can be difficult to wash your hands. You may be away from a bathroom, or accidentally touch something *after* washing your hands. For that reason, I carry hand sanitizer everywhere I go. I carry it in my purse and in my car and have it sitting in my kitchen and on my desk at work. I recommend you do the same. Use it, and use it often.

The Role of Supplements

Ms. Catherine came to her appointment armed with a list of questions. Recently diagnosed with stage 2 triple negative breast cancer, the 60-year-old woman refused to receive chemotherapy after resection of her breast cancer. "I just don't think I could handle chemo," she said. "It's too toxic. I'd prefer to do something natural." She looked at me over her stack of papers. "What supplements can I take to make sure the cancer doesn't come back?"

Supplements are everywhere—pills to help you lose weight, pills to help you fall asleep, and pills to help you enhance certain body parts. Go online, and you will find websites touting the ability of different supplements to heal every ailment known to man, from toenail fungus to cancer. What is real and what is not?

Unfortunately, we do not know the answer to that question. Typically, when a drug is manufactured, it goes through rigorous testing to determine if it has the desired outcome. However, supplements are not subjected to the same rigorous tests that are applied to pharmaceutical drugs. Sure, they can be tested in mice and rats, but there are many differences between mice and men.

If you are interested in using a particular supplement, I recommend you research the supplement and discuss it with your oncologist. Your oncologist will look the supplement up to make sure that there are no major interactions with your treatment. Ninety-nine percent of the time, your doctor will tell you the supplement is fine to take. If the supplement actually helps you, that's wonderful. Even if it does not do anything, it will help you gain a sense of control over your treatment, as well as a sense of participation. That can be just as powerful as a prescribed pill.

What about Ms. Catherine's question? What supplements can you take to improve your chances of being cancer free?

No one has an answer to that question, unfortunately. But we call them supplements for a reason. They should be taken to *supplement* your treatment, not replace your treatment. You will never find a head to head trial where one hundred people with cancer were randomized to receive either chemotherapy or a nutritional supplement. In the absence of that data, I will never tell you to take a supplement in place of tried and true treatment.

Having discussed the lack of evidence to show the benefits of most supplements, there *are* some supplements that make more sense to me than others. The supplements that I would support are listed below. Of course, you should discuss any supplement you plan on taking with your oncologist first. Everyone is different—what is fine for one person could be harmful to you. However, in general, these supplements are benign and there is enough data to suggest that they could be of *some* benefit. For dosing, you can look on WebMD or go to your nearest vitamin shop.

Examples of Some Beneficial Supplements	
Turmeric	Reported to have anti-inflammatory effects.
Pomegranate juice	High in antioxidants, which protect cells from something known as "free radicals." Free radicals can cause mutations in your DNA, leading to the development of cancer cells.

Sesame seed oil	Anecdotally reported to help improve thrombocytopenia.
Green tea	High in antioxidants. Can stimulate metabolism.
Cinnamon	Reported to lower blood sugar, also possibly has antioxidant effects.
Melatonin	Studies have shown it can help regulate day and night cycles, which can improve insomnia.
Vitamin B12	Low vitamin B12 levels can result in anemia and fatigue.

There are also some supplements that I would *not* take unless absolutely necessary, and even then should only be taken under the monitoring of a physician. These supplements are listed below. If you feel strongly that these supplements would help you, please discuss them further with your cancer doctor.

Examples of Some Potentially Harmful Supplements	
Estrogen	Can be found in many supplements for menopause, including red clover, flaxseed, and black cohosh. Estrogen use can be potentially dangerous for women diagnosed with breast cancer, and can potentially even increase your risk for developing breast cancer.
Testosterone	Can be found in many supplements promoting "virility" for men. Be cautious— testosterone can be dangerous for men diagnosed with prostate cancer.

℟ The Role of Complementary Medicine

"Is it ok for me to have a massage?" Mr. George asked. Aside from stage 4 prostate cancer, Mr. George was in fairly good health. However, he suffered from chronic back pain unrelated to his cancer. "My back has really been giving me fits."

As I've mentioned, most complementary medicine is fine with me. For the majority of my patients, massage is a great way to relax and improve circulation.[16] Ask your oncologist what regions the masseuse should avoid, and then convey that to your masseuse. I am also a supporter of acupuncture. I think that acupuncture can do wonders for pain and neuropathy caused by chemotherapy. Unfortunately, most complementary medicine will not be covered by your insurance. However, if you can afford it, I think complementary medicine is a great addition to your traditional treatment.

"What about CBD oil?" you ask.

CBD oil, or **cannobidiol oil**, is an extract of cannabis or marijuana plants. It has recently become very popular for the treatment of a variety of disorders, from epilepsy to depression to arthritis. If you go on the internet and search for "CBD" and "cancer," you will find hundreds, if not thousands, of websites discussing the potential benefits of CBD oil for cancer patients. Is any of it real?

---

[16] If you have been diagnosed with bone metastases, or cancer that has spread to the bone, ask your oncologist if massage is safe for you. Most likely, your oncologist will tell you specific areas you masseuse should avoid, and you can pass that information on to your masseuse.

At this time, we have low-quality evidence to suggest that CBD oil has any significant anti-cancer effects in humans. While there have been many studies evaluating its role in relieving specific chemotherapy side effects, none of the studies have shown strong enough evidence to convince the FDA or the NCCN that CBD oil should be recommended or approved for specific cancer care use. Because of this, your insurance company will not pay for CBD oil or medical marijuana, and these treatments can get very expensive.

Please discuss using CBD oil and medical marijuana with your oncologist. Personally, for most of my own patients, I do not mind if they use CBD oil or medical marijuana. While there is no proof that it helps, at the end of the day, if you feel that CBD oil or medical marijuana helps you, then it is fine with me. Whatever helps you to feel better during chemotherapy helps me do my job as your cancer doctor.

That being said, I would advise against *smoking* medical marijuana. Marijuana is a plant and can develop mold when it is in the process of being dried. If you smoke the marijuana, this mold can get into your lungs. Normally, when your immune system is intact, that is not a big issue. However, while on chemotherapy, your immune system will be suppressed and smoking marijuana can possibly lead to a fungal lung infection.

If you are interested in pursuing medical marijuana, inform your oncologist. Most likely he or she will have contact information for someone who performs medical marijuana certifications. After you obtain your medical marijuana certification, which will likely cost around $100-150 in cash, you will need to bring your certification to a dispensary. The dispensary will prescribe and provide your medical marijuana for an additional cash charge.

Please note that while medical marijuana is legal in some states, it is not legal in every state in the U.S. Additionally, while medical marijuana may be legal in some states, it is still against federal law. It is a felony offense to transport marijuana across state lines, even if the person doing so is an approved medical marijuana patient. Similar laws apply to transporting marijuana by airplane.

If you choose to use medical marijuana, be smart, and be safe. First, discuss using medical marijuana with your oncologist. Do not use medical marijuana before driving or operating machinery. Do not transport your medical marijuana across state lines. Do not leave it where someone other than the prescribed individual can intentionally or accidentally use it, and keep it away from children and pets.

WHAT YOU HAVE LEARNED IN THIS SECTION

Summary:

- If you are struggling with nausea or decreased appetite, I prefer calories over content. Eat whatever appeals to you.
- If you are eating well and having no issues with maintaining your weight, I recommend a high protein, low sugar diet that is rich in antioxidants.

- If you are currently receiving chemotherapy, please stop losing weight. *After* chemotherapy or if you are taking a medication that causes weight gain, I recommend the Pink Ribbon Diet for weight management.
- Stay hydrated and wash your hands.
- Most supplements and forms of complementary medicine are fine. However, please discuss with your oncologist prior to starting any new health regimen.

In this section, I have provided information about diet and weight management. In addition, I have provided information regarding the role of supplements and complementary medicine. Please remember that though I am a doctor, I am not *your* doctor. The information provided in this section is intended for educational purposes and not meant to treat any medical conditions. Please discuss all changes in your medications, diet, and exercise with your oncologist.

In the next section, I will discuss some common frustrations patients express when hospitalized. Though some patients will never require hospitalization throughout their chemotherapy, many do end up admitted to the hospital for some reason or another during their treatment. In the next section, I will provide some insight as to what happens "behind the scenes" when it comes to your inpatient hospital care.

Hospitalizations

On Monday morning, I logged onto my hospital computer as usual. I pulled up my inpatient hospital list and scanned it for names that I recognized. I always checked the list prior to starting clinic to see if any of my patients were currently admitted to the hospital.

To my surprise, Ms. Elizabeth's name popped up on my census. I quickly scanned her chart. It looked like she was hospitalized for cellulitis, or a skin infection, of her left foot. She had just completed her tenth week of chemotherapy last week.

I went over to the hospital and found her room. "Knock, knock," I said, walking through the open door. "Good morning."

"Dr. DeRidder!" she exclaimed. Ms. Elizabeth was sitting on her hospital bed with her left foot propped up on pillows. She gestured to her foot, which was covered with gauze. "Can you believe it?"

"What happened?" I asked. "You were doing great last week!"

"I know!" She shook her head with frustration. "Gerry and I were walking our dog, Suzie, and it was getting dark. She got spooked by something and started pulling at her leash. I lost my balance and took a step forward, and somehow bashed my toe against the curb." She sighed. "I was wearing sandals so it got pretty scraped up. A couple of days later it started getting red, and then yesterday I noticed pus around the nail. Gerry made me go to the emergency room, and I guess they thought I needed to stay."

I took a look at her foot. Like she had said, her big toe was swollen and discolored. "Well, I think you made the right call," I told her. "The last thing we'd want is for the infection to get out of hand."

"I know," she said. "I think I made the right call too." She hesitated. "I am a little confused though." She gestured to her foot. "When I first came to the emergency room, one of the nurses mentioned that I might need to have a scan done to see if there's a blood clot in my leg since my ankle is swollen. A couple of hours later, though, the doctor said it wasn't necessary. No one has mentioned it since. Is that normal?"

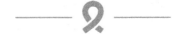

I hope that you or your loved one is never sick enough to require hospitalization. That being said, many patients diagnosed with cancer do require hospitalization at some point, whether it is for symptoms from their cancer, side effects from their chemotherapy, or like, Ms. Elizabeth, for something completely unrelated to their cancer care. For most patients, their introduction to the inpatient medical setting can be confusing and chaotic, and they can be left with more questions than answers. Much like Ms. Elizabeth's experience, different members of your health care team may tell you different, and sometimes conflicting, things.

The purpose of this section is to review a couple of common issues that arise in the inpatient medical world. My hope is that the information in this chapter will provide you a "sneak peek" into what happens behind the scenes as your doctors work to get you back on your feet.

WHAT YOU WILL GET OUT OF THIS SECTION

Every doctor is telling me something different	Why your diagnosis and treatment keeps changing while you are in the hospital.
Medicine is both an art and a science	A reminder that much about the human body remains a mystery.

℞ *Every Doctor Is Telling Me Something Different*

If you or a loved one has ever been hospitalized, you may already know what I am talking about. The moment you walked into the hospital, you likely had doctors telling you different—and sometimes contradicting—things. One doctor might have told you that you had pneumonia. Two days later, another doctor may have told you that actually, you might have pneumonia, but you might also have cancer. One week later, you were told you definitely have cancer, and that you probably never had pneumonia to begin with.

"Why is every doctor telling me something different?" you wonder.

Unfortunately, this is a very common phenomenon. When someone first comes to the hospital, doctors are trying to make a diagnosis. We piece together the story based on your medical history, your symptoms, the timeline, your vital signs, imaging, and labs. Each data point is another part of the story. As we gather more data points, our opinions can change.

In this manner, making a medical diagnosis is similar to assembling a 1,000 piece puzzle. At first, all we have are a couple of corner pieces. Piece by piece, we add to the puzzle. As we do so, we are required to guess what the picture shows. *I think this is a picture of a kitten,* one person thinks. We add some more puzzle pieces. We see a long whisker, a long piece of a tail. *Hmmm,* someone else thinks, *maybe this is actually a cat.* We spend hours putting together the background, trying to shift through unimportant pieces and the pieces that are actually necessary. Finally, we find a piece of a paw, a tawny mane, and an ear. Lo and behold—we have been looking at a lion all along.

As doctors, we are trying to put together one of the most mysterious puzzles ever created: the human body. When you are admitted to the hospital, all we are given are a couple of puzzle pieces. We painfully try to reconstruct the picture. Along the way, we are required to guess what the picture shows. We do our best. We look at the pieces we have and try to fill in the rest of the picture. As we gain more and more pieces, our guesses get better and better. However, that also means our guesses sometimes change. Sometimes, as we put the puzzle together, pieces that we thought were important turn out to be background picture. Sometimes pieces that we thought were background turn out to be vital.

I know it can be extremely frustrating. One day you are told one thing, and the next, something else. Remember that we are trying our best.

MS. KYLE'S STORY

Ms. Kyle was a 62-year-old woman with tongue cancer that had been treated with a combination of chemotherapy and radiation. She finished her therapy and overall did very well. However, her post-treatment scan showed that there was a 3.5cm mass still sitting at the back of her tongue. Her ear, nose, and throat doctor and I both recommended that she have the mass biopsied. However, Ms. Kyle refused. She had just made it through the ordeal of chemoradiation. She wanted to take a month off and then come back for the biopsy.

Fast forward to six weeks later. I received a call from an ICU physician. Ms. Kyle was in the hospital with an overwhelming blood infection. She had significant swelling around her throat, and a CT scan showed that in addition to the mass behind her tongue, she now had a new abscess in her throat.

The next day, I went to see her in the ICU, where I talked to her distraught wife. "I looked over her scan," I told her. "To me, this looks like she has a pretty severe infection."

"What?" her wife exclaimed. "They told me that it's her cancer causing her to be sick."

I shook my head. I had looked over her most recent CT scan and it was highly suspicious for an infection. "Perhaps they thought that before," I replied, "but her most recent CT scan is pretty convincing for an abscess."

"I don't understand," her wife said with frustration. "They said it was the cancer before. But now it's an infection?" She looked over at her critically ill wife with tears in her eyes. "Every doctor is telling me something different. Why can't you all get together and agree on what's going on?"

Sometimes, each doctor has a different opinion as to what the puzzle shows. As doctors, we have specialties. When we look at the puzzle pieces, we are looking at them through a filter of our specialty. You have probably heard the saying "When you're a hammer, everything looks like a nail." The same thing applies to medicine. When you are a cancer doctor, everything could be cancer. If you are an infectious disease doctor, everything could be an infection. We are each looking at the puzzle, and interpreting it within the context of our own expertise.

Ms. Kyle's wife's question was a good one. Can we all get together and agree on what is going on?

We *do* communicate with each other. We *do* call one another and talk over scenarios. However, in each hospital, there are hundreds up to thousands of patients admitted each day. Trying to coordinate multidisciplinary physician gatherings for every patient can be difficult, if not impossible. The process is certainly not perfect, but we are trying. Please be patient with us.

The puzzle takes time to put together.

Medicine Is Both an Art and a Science

As doctors, we study information in books, we do trials, and we focus on numbers and data. This makes sense because medicine is considered a science. However, there is another side to medicine, one that cannot be found on paper and computer screens. This side is known as "the art" of medicine.

When I approach the treatment of an illness, I base my decisions on a loose set of premises. If you have an infection, and I know what type of infection, I can make a reasonable guess as to what type of antibiotic I should prescribe. My decision is based on science. I know which types of antibiotics treat which particular infections based on prior scientific studies. In addition to what medicine is most effective for treating your infection, however, there are multiple other considerations that need to be taken into account. Do you have any allergies? Do you have any other medical conditions that can interact with the antibiotic? How many days of antibiotics should I give?

Here is where the art of medicine comes into play. Experience, conscientiousness, and intuition all play a role when I choose which antibiotic to prescribe. If you ask three different physicians which antibiotic he or she would prescribe, you might get a different type of antibiotic, dose, and duration from each physician. Is one better than the other? Not necessarily. However, the side effects and overall patient experience may differ depending on which medication is prescribed. The art of medicine is figuring out which medicine works best for which patient.

The same concept applies to your cancer care. When I start a patient on chemotherapy, I go by standard treatment recommendations provided by the National Comprehensive Cancer Network (NCCN). However, as we proceed with your treatment, my role as your oncologist is to adjust your therapy based on the feedback your body is giving me. The adjustments that I make are based partly on science, experience, and intuition. The adjustments I choose might be slightly different compared to one of my colleagues. Ultimately, the goal is the same—to keep you healthy and treat your cancer.

Because medicine is both an art and a science, it can make results harder to predict, especially if you focus too hard on numbers.

MS. ESTHER'S STORY

Ms. Esther was an 88-year-old woman referred to my office for thrombocytopenia. I diagnosed her with Idiopathic Thrombocytopenia Purpura (ITP). She received weekly shots of N-plate, a medication designed to stimulate production of platelets. Her son was an engineer, and very interested in her treatment. One day, as we sat down for a follow up appointment, he pulled out a line chart that he had made of her platelet counts over the past month.

"She received 1mcg/kg of the medication three weeks ago," he said, "and her platelet count didn't budge. So you increased it to 2mcg/kg, and her platelet count went from 11 to 21. But when you increased it to 3mcg/kg, her platelet count went from 21 to 88. Is that normal? How much will each increase in dose increase her platelet count? Is it a linear increase or exponential?"

I smiled at Ms. Esther's son. "That's a great question. Unfortunately, I can't answer it. The body does what the body wants. There is no way to know how much her platelet count will jump with the increased dose. We just increase until her platelet count goes above 50, and then we keep her at that dose. Even with that dose, it's completely normal for the count to fluctuate. One week her platelet count will be 100, the next 60, the next 80. It doesn't mean the medication is not working—the fluctuation is a normal part of the process."

I could tell that he was frustrated by my answer, and I understood his frustration. As humans, we want to see linear progress in the right direction. We want to be able to plot out the numbers, and say, "If I put X in the equation, it will solve for Y."

In the field of medicine, however, oftentimes we cannot do that. Sometimes we give a medication and it does not work, though all indications suggest that it should work perfectly. We might never understand why it does not work. Sometimes we give a medication as a last-ditch effort, a "Hail Mary pass" of sorts, and it miraculously works. Why did it work? We might never know.

At the end of the day, we base our decisions on science, and we use science to adjust our treatments. However, sometimes the body defies our explanations.

Because medicine is both an art and a science, it can make results harder to predict, especially if you focus too hard on numbers. My recommendation is to focus on the big picture and the overall trends. Remember that you are a human and not a robot. I cannot type a set of commands into your keyboard and have your body spit out information exactly as predicted. Try not to get too caught up in the numbers, because they can fluctuate. This is especially true in the inpatient setting, where we are often checking your labs on a daily basis. If your numbers go up or go down, do not panic. Remember that medicine is an art and a science. Sometimes with art, you have to take a step back from the picture to see all the pieces come together. So take a deep breath, and take a step back.

WHAT YOU HAVE LEARNED IN THIS SECTION

Summary:

- During your hospitalization, our diagnoses and treatments will often change based on the feedback your body provides us.
- Every doctor has a unique approach to medicine. Every patient has a slightly different response to treatment.
- We are only beginning to understand the complexity of the human body.

In this section, I have reviewed common issues patients struggle with while in the hospital. I discussed why your doctors might be giving you different answers on an almost daily basis. I also reviewed why it is important to realize that medicine is both an art and a science. No two doctors will approach a problem from exactly the same angle, and the results you get may not be linear or expected. However, the ultimate goal of everyone on your inpatient team is to get you feeling better and back home.

This section concludes Chapter 5. If you have made it this far in your reading, congratulations! My hope is that with the knowledge you have gained, you will thrive during your chemotherapy. Soon, you will be able to look back and say, "I did it. I am a cancer survivor."

In the next chapter, I will briefly discuss what happens *after* completing chemotherapy.The following chapter is brief for a reason; your cancer surveillance plan depends heavily on the type and stage of your cancer.

CHAPTER 6

Survivorship

"Congratulations!" I said to Ms. Elizabeth as I walked into the room. "Last day of chemo!"

She beamed at me. She was here for her last dose of weekly chemotherapy. "I know," she said. "I'm so happy." Her husband sitting next to her smiled and squeezed her hand.

"So what happens next?" she asked.

"Well, after this you need to meet with your radiation doctor. If you remember from when you first met with him a couple of months ago, he had recommended six weeks of radiation after you finished your chemo." She nodded.

"My office will call over to let the radiation doctor know that you've finished chemo, and they'll get you plugged in to start your radiation in the next couple of weeks. Two weeks after you finish radiation, I'll start you on a pill that will help to reduce your risk of cancer coming back over the next 5-10 years."

For the next ten minutes, we talked more about the medication and possible side effects. "After you finish radiation," I concluded, "you'll stay on this pill for at least five years. I'll have you come back to see me every three months for the first year, and then we'll space out our visits after that."

"What about scans?" she asked.

"Well, we recommend that you have a yearly mammogram. However, aside from that, the national guidelines recommend against doing routine CT scans or PET scans as part of the follow up for patients with early stage breast cancer."

As I wrapped up our appointment, I could tell she was getting emotional. "What's wrong?" I asked.

"I can't believe I made it," she said. "I mean, I know that I had it easy compared to what some patients have been through. But it was still really tough. I just wanted to say thank you for taking such good care of me." She wiped her eyes. "I can't believe it's my turn to ring the bell!" Downstairs in our infusion center, there was a bell that patients could ring on their last day of treatment.

"It's been a pleasure, dear." I stood and gave her a hug. "You've done fantastic. Now go downstairs and ring that bell."

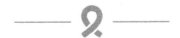

After you complete chemotherapy, like Ms. Elizabeth, you will enter a phase known as "surveillance" or **"survivorship."**

With most cancers, the highest risk of recurrence is within the first five years. Therefore, for the first five years after your cancer treatment, your doctors will be monitoring you closely to make sure there are no signs or symptoms of your cancer returning. Each cancer and stage typically has a different "surveillance" plan. Once you complete your cancer treatment, your oncologist will talk to you about what your specific surveillance plan will entail. Your surveillance follow up appointments will typically consist of labs, possibly imaging, and a physical examination performed by your oncologist. The National Cancer Institute has published a very helpful guide to survivorship called, *Facing Forward: Life After Cancer Treatment*. You can find this free booklet online as a PDF or download it to your e-reader.

Since your survivorship plan depends on your cancer type, stage, and form of chemotherapy, what applies to one patient may not apply to another. For that reason, I will not go in-depth into the many issues that surround survivorship. However, no matter what type of cancer you had or what type of treatment you received, one tenet remains true. *You have to follow up with your cancer doctor after completing treatment.*

Why? Well, once you finish chemotherapy, you may need additional phases of cancer treatment. Like Ms. Elizabeth, you may need radiation or other forms of treatment such as endocrine therapy or surgery. Your medical oncologist will help to coordinate your care so that you don't "fall through the cracks" of the medical system.

In addition, you just received multiple doses of heavy-duty chemicals designed to kill cancer cells. All chemotherapy has side effects. Your cancer doctor should have discussed these potential side effects with you before you received your first dose of treatment. However, sometimes patients can have prolonged or delayed side effects, such as neuropathy, or numbness and tingling in the fingers and toes. While these side effects may get better on their own, they may need special monitoring or treatment.

Finally, unfortunately, despite everything you've been through, cancer can come back. Depending on your cancer type, it can come back within months, or it can come back within years. Your cancer doctor knows what symptoms and signs to look out for, as well as whether or not you need scans to monitor for cancer recurrence. If you had surgery and/or radiation, you will also need to follow up with your surgeon and/or radiation oncologist.

WHAT YOU HAVE LEARNED IN THIS CHAPTER

Summary:

- After you complete your treatment, you will enter a phase known as "surveillance" or "survivorship."
- Each cancer type and stage has a different type of survivorship plan.
- Please continue to follow up with your oncologist after you complete your cancer treatment.

If you have reached this point in your treatment, congratulations! If you have just started your cancer journey, don't worry. You'll get there eventually. Know that you are strong, smart, and have power over your cancer treatment choices. By reading this book, you are giving yourself the knowledge you need to do well.

The following chapter is titled, "*Chapter 7: Stage 4 Cancer.*" Up until now, this book has focused on issues pertinent to patients with early stage, curable cancer. Some of these issues also apply to patients with advanced, incurable cancers. However, there are some topics that are unique to patients with advanced cancer. If you were diagnosed with stage 4 or incurable cancer, please read on. The next chapter is for you. If you have early stage cancer, feel free to either continue reading or to flip ahead to the section labeled "*Conclusions.*"

CHAPTER 7

Stage 4 Cancer

Ms. Elizabeth sat in my office again, this time next to her friend, Ms. Pat. Ms. Pat was a 53-year-old woman recently diagnosed with stage 4 colon cancer. She had received her diagnosis and started treatment at another hospital, but was not happy with the care she had been receiving. Today was our first appointment together.

"Hi there," I introduced myself. "As you know, I'm Dr. DeRidder. I've looked through your records so I have an understanding of what's been going on. I'm just going to go through what my understanding is of the situation, and fill me in if there is anything that I missed." Ms. Pat nodded.

Quickly I summarized Ms. Pat's history. She had been diagnosed with colon cancer approximately 4 months ago. She had gone to her primary care doctor for belly pain and had a scan of her abdomen performed. Unfortunately, the scan of her belly showed multiple masses in her liver and her lungs. A liver biopsy revealed colon cancer.

"So your oncologist started you on a type of chemotherapy known as FOLFOX," I concluded. "You've been receiving this for about 3 months, and it sounds like overall you've done well, though things have been a little bumpy."

She nodded. "Yeah...it's been tough. A lot of fatigue, just feeling really run down. It's hard because my husband also has health issues, so a lot of the housekeeping and cooking falls on me. I kept telling my doctor, and I just felt like he wasn't listening to me."

I nodded. "Sure. Well, I always say, let's start at the beginning. I'm just going to review some of the basics. A lot of this you probably already know."

Unfortunately, it became quickly clear that a lot of the information Ms. Pat did not already know.

"...once cancer has gone from one organ to another, it's typically considered stage 4 cancer," I said. "So because your cancer has gone from the colon to the liver and lungs, you have a stage 4 colon cancer."

I looked at Ms. Pat's face. She looked shell shocked.

"Is this new information? Did your doctor not tell you this?"

She shook her head. "No! I mean...no, not at all! He said that it was in my liver and lungs, but he didn't say anything about being stage 4! I mean, what, what..." She burst into tears. Ms. Elizabeth wrapped her arms around her.

"I'm so sorry," I said. "I'm not sure why your doctor didn't tell you."

"So...so what do we do?" she asked.

"Well...we know that the way cancer gets from one organ to another is through the blood system," I continued. "A piece of cancer cell will break off and travel through the blood system, using it like a highway. This is how your cancer got from your colon to your liver and your lungs.

"Knowing this is important because it dictates how we treat the cancer. Because the cancer is in your blood system, we have to give you a treatment that also goes through your blood system—chemotherapy."

I continued on, talking about the chemotherapy she had received in the past, and my plans for chemotherapy moving forward. Finally, I stopped. If her doctor had not told her about her cancer stage, he probably had not told her about her prognosis either.

"One thing that I discuss with all my patients is prognosis, or how long you have to live. Is that something that you want to know about, or would you rather not know?"

Ms. Pat looked at Ms. Elizabeth. Ms. Elizabeth shook her head. "I can't answer that for you."

"I want to know," Ms. Pat said.

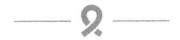

If you have been diagnosed with stage 4 cancer, it means that like Ms. Pat, your cancer involves more than one organ. For instance, a stage 4 cancer would be a breast cancer that has spread from the breast to the liver, or a prostate cancer that has spread from the prostate to the bone. As I discussed with Ms. Pat, knowing your cancer stage is vital to creating your treatment plan. We know the way your cancer spread was through the blood system. A cancer cell broke off from the original tumor and traveled through the blood system, using it like a highway.

Surgery and radiation are both considered local treatments, meaning that they touch only one area of your body. However, if cancer has entered into your blood system, I know that cancer cells can potentially travel anywhere. With that in mind, I need to treat you with something that *can go anywhere the cancer can go.* Typically, that means chemotherapy.

Like I told Ms. Pat, chemotherapy often remains the cornerstone of treatment for stage 4 cancer. However, the goal of chemotherapy is different for stage 4 cancer compared to earlier cancer stages. With stage 4 cancer, while chemotherapy can potentially control and even shrink your cancer, typically it cannot get rid of your cancer forever. Why? Because the amount of chemotherapy needed to kill every single cancer cell in the blood system would be too toxic for the human body to tolerate.

This means that while I can attempt to slow down your cancer and improve your quality of life, the majority of the time, I cannot cure your cancer.[17]

I am sorry. I wish that our treatments were better. I wish that we had the technology and medicine to have prevented your cancer from occurring in the first place. You are entitled to feel anger, hurt, betrayal, and fear. However, you are not alone in this fight. In this chapter, I will discuss how to live with a stage 4 cancer diagnosis, and important concepts to understand as you initiate treatment. Your cancer doctor is here to support you.

If you skipped ahead to this chapter, finish this chapter, but afterward, please go back and read Chapter 2 through 5. Most of the information contained within those chapters will apply to you as well.

WHAT YOU WILL GET OUT OF THIS CHAPTER

Finding a new normal with stage 4 cancer	A reminder that though your life has changed, *you* control your attitude towards these changes.
Chemotherapy cannot restore health	A discussion about the limits of what chemotherapy can achieve.

[17] There are some rare exceptions to this statement. Please discuss with your oncologist your stage and your prognosis.

Quality of life	A discussion about the goals of chemotherapy with stage 4 cancer.
It Is okay to say "No" to treatment	A reminder that you are the captain of this ship.
The role of palliative care	An explanation about the role of palliative care.
Hospice does not mean giving up	A discussion about the role of hospice.
There is always hope	A reminder that there is always, always hope.

🎗 *Finding a New Normal With Stage 4 Cancer*

As mentioned, stage 4 cancer can be controlled, even de-creased in size—but it typically cannot be cured. This means that for most individuals diagnosed with stage 4 cancer, you will need to remain on chemotherapy or some type of medication indefinitely. With that being said, it is important to realize that you may never be able to return completely to your pre-cancer life. Some of the activities you used to enjoy, you might not be able to do anymore.

However, while chemotherapy may not be able to restore you to the person that you once were, it can give you more time. Time to spend with family—time to remember and reflect. Time to enjoy quieter, simpler moments. You may not be able to go for a mile hike in the park. However, you can still sit outside and enjoy the sunshine. You can still walk around your neigh-borhood. There is still so much joy that can be gained from life.

MR. ROBERT'S STORY

Mr. Robert was a 39-year-old man diagnosed with acute leukemia. He was admitted to the hospital for over six weeks to receive high dose chemotherapy in an attempt to treat his leukemia. His immune system was dramatically suppressed because of his chemo-therapy, but eventually, his immune system improved and he was able to be discharged home. Despite ex-tensive education about neutropenic precautions, he decided to go crabbing in the Chesapeake Bay. Prior to his diagnosis, he was a waterman, and crabbing was one of the activities he had enjoyed most during the summer.

One warm summer day, he spent six hours out on his boat and went crabbing in the Chesapeake Bay barefoot. Two days later he was admitted to the hospital with severe skin infections in both legs. He ended up remaining in the hospital for almost a month being treated for his infections.

The hospitalization served as a wake-up call for Mr. Robert. Life was different since his cancer diagnosis, and his body was not the same as it was before. He learned that if he wanted to be around for his two-year-old daughter, he had to change his habits as well as his hobbies. His crabbing days were over. Nowadays, he enjoys spending time sitting on the dock, teaching his daughter how to fish.

You will need to acknowledge how cancer has impacted your life—and accept the changes. If you keep thinking, "Once I get better, I'll be able to X, Y, Z...," you will have a difficult journey ahead of you. The reason for this is that chemotherapy *rarely* ever makes anyone feel better. Chemotherapy can stabilize. It can shrink tumors. However, rarely will it ever restore health. Of course, there are rare exceptions to this statement. However, as a whole, if you have been diagnosed with stage 4 cancer, you will need to accept that your life has been irrevocably changed.

Of course, it is okay to lament or mourn what you have lost. However, you will need to discover a "new normal." Otherwise, you will spend whatever time God and chemotherapy can give you depressed and anxious. Instead, think about the things you used to enjoy. Then think about what you can still do. Let go of the old, and embrace your current life. While there is so much in your life right now that you cannot control, you *can* control how you approach your diagnosis and what you do with your life now. Establish a "new normal" and move forward. Accept that things might never be the same again—but there are still a lot of things worth living for.

Chemotherapy Cannot Restore Health[18]

Surprisingly, it is a very common misconception that chemotherapy can restore health. I have often heard well-meaning family members tell loved ones, "The chemotherapy is going to help you get stronger," or "The chemotherapy is going to make you better." Part of this misconception comes from hope, part from fear, and part from a desire to protect your loved one from further pain.

The truth is, with stage 4 cancer, chemotherapy *can* stabilize your health and prevent it from getting worse. However, it cannot reverse time. It cannot restore you to the person that you were a year ago, as much as I wish it could.

---

[18] Of course, every patient is different, and there can be exceptions to this statement, particularly with leukemia and lymphoma.

I think of using chemotherapy like using superglue to repair a much loved, but broken lamp. If the lamp is broken, the glue will keep the parts together and help the lamp function. However, the glue does not change the fact that the lamp was broken to begin with—and that at some point in the future, the lamp will likely break again.

Similarly, if you have cancer, it has irrevocably changed your body. Most patients with stage 4 cancer have some type of cancer symptoms. We use modern medicine to relieve these symptoms as best we can and to enable your body to function again. Then, we give chemotherapy to stabilize your cancer. Chemotherapy can potentially keep your cancer in check. However, chemotherapy will never completely heal what is already broken. Chemotherapy will not make you stronger or heal the symptoms that you already have. At best, it will stabilize your health and keep your symptoms from getting worse as long as possible.

MR. JOB'S STORY

Mr. Job was a 79-year-old man who lived by himself with no family in the local area. One night, he was brought to the hospital by his daughter, who came to visit from out of state and found him unconscious in his home. His labs showed that his kidneys had shut down. Imaging revealed that in addition to cancer in his bones, Mr. Job had a 12cm bladder mass that was blocking the flow of urine from his kidneys to his bladder.

To relieve this blockage, tubes were placed into his kidneys. The tubes emptied into bags taped to his back. With the blockage removed, his kidneys began to work and he began to improve. At that point, I was called to see him and discuss his cancer treatment.

I met with Mr. Job at his bedside. That afternoon, I discussed with him and his daughter that he had stage 4 bladder cancer and that his cancer was not curable. However, now that his kidneys were working better, and he was feeling better, he would be a candidate for immunotherapy. The goal of his immunotherapy would be to try to shrink or stabilize his cancer.

"You see, dad," his daughter said. "You can get the treatment, and then the bags can come off."

"Well," I told his daughter, "not exactly."

The goal of Mr. Job's immunotherapy would be to prevent his cancer from getting worse. Unfortunately, immunotherapy would most likely *not* shrink his cancer to the point that his kidney tubes could be removed. In short, while I hoped to stabilize his condition, it was unlikely that his health or his body would completely return to normal.

This news was hard for Mr. Job to hear. That being said, it was important for him to know the truth.

A year later, though he still has urine bags taped to his back, he is feeling well, eating, and enjoying time with his granddaughter. He is living life to the fullest because he knows that at some point, his life is going to end. He understands that though we always hope for cancer to disappear, most of the time it will not. Most of the time, the most we can hope for is "stable disease."

At the end of the day, the goal is to shrink the cancer as much as possible, as long as possible, and to make whatever time God gives you as good as possible. With that in mind, it is important to understand your disease, the goals of your treatment, and the limitations of your treatment.

Quality of Life

In medicine, "**quality of life**" is used to describe the health, comfort, and happiness experienced by an individual. In oncology, quality of life is extremely important. For patients with stage 4 cancer, some might say that quality of life is everything.

If you have been diagnosed with stage 4 cancer, by now you know that most likely your cancer is not curable. So if I cannot cure your cancer, what is my goal with your treatment?

There are two main goals. First, my goal is to shrink the cancer as much as possible, and as long as possible. I hope to give you as much time as I can on this earth. More importantly, however, my goal is to make sure that whatever time you have left is as good as possible. As I mentioned earlier, chemotherapy cannot *improve* your health, but it can *stabilize* your health. The goal with chemotherapy in stage 4 cancer is to prevent your symptoms from worsening and to prevent new symptoms. The goal is to make whatever time God gives you as good as possible so that you can do the things that you want to do—spend time with loved ones, achieve dreams, and do hobbies that you have always enjoyed. The goal with chemotherapy in stage 4 cancer is to improve *length* of life as well as *quality* of life.

Almost all patients worry about quality of life. I have had many patients tell me, "If the chemotherapy can't cure me, I don't want chemotherapy. I don't want to be sick from side effects in the last years or months of my life."

I assure patients that I completely understand. If I cannot cure your cancer, the last thing I *ever* want to do is rob you of whatever time you have left. My job as an oncologist is to pick an appropriate chemotherapy or medication for you, adjust the dose, and manage your side effects. By taking into account your performance status, your cancer, and your other health issues, I should be able to appropriately treat your cancer while still preserving your quality of life.

What if your performance status is not strong enough for chemotherapy? What if your performance status worsens while receiving chemotherapy? Well, that's when we sit down and talk. That's when we go over your goals of care and talk about whether chemotherapy is still your best option.

What if *you* think you're not strong enough for chemotherapy?

When we start chemotherapy, you are not signing a contract. If at any point you think that your quality of life is now worse because of my treatment, all you need to do is tell me. It's your life and it's your body—you always have the right to say no more treatment.

Ultimately, talk to your doctor about your goals for your treatment. If your treatment goal is quality of life, *tell your doctor*. If your goal is quantity of life above all else, again, *tell your doctor*. Only by understanding your priorities can your oncologist create a treatment plan that will achieve your goals and meet your needs.

It Is Okay to Say "No" to Treatment

I encourage you to go to your oncology appointment, hear your options, and hear about treatment benefits and risks. If you decide you want to move forward with cancer treatment, that's your decision. If you decide against treatment, that's also your decision. If at any point you do not feel comfortable proceeding, you can say "Stop!" and that's *definitely* your decision! Furthermore, I will respect that choice. As your cancer doctor, my job is simply to present to you the treatment options available, and the risks and benefits of those options. I may give you my opinion as to which treatment option I would recommend. However, after that, how we move forward is completely up to you.

MR. EDWIN'S STORY

Mr. Edwin was an 89-year-old man with newly diagnosed stage 4 prostate cancer. As I walked into the room and introduced myself, I noticed that he looked extremely nervous. I sat down and did my usual discussion about his cancer diagnosis and stage.

When I started talking about his treatment options, I saw the anxiety on his face ratchet up. Finally, I had to stop. "What's wrong, Mr. Edwin?" I asked.

"Do I need chemotherapy?" he responded.

"Actually, no," I said. "We can give you a shot that will lower your testosterone levels, and essentially remove your cancer's food supply. The cancer will shrink, and your biggest side effect will be hot flashes."

The flood of relief on his face was immediate. "Oh, I'm so glad," he said. "My wife died from breast cancer forty years ago. I always said that if I needed chemotherapy, I wasn't going to do it. I almost didn't come today."

"I'm sorry to hear about your wife," I responded, "and I'm glad that we have another option than chemotherapy for you. But even if I had said that you did need chemotherapy, you always have the right to say no! It's your body and your life. No one is going to force you to do anything."

At the end of the day, living with cancer is like trying to sail a ship through stormy seas. The weather is blinding, the waters choppy, and you can easily lose your sense of direction. It is easy to feel like you are being tossed this way and that way, with no control over the situation. However, you are the captain of this ship. You are at the steering wheel, and you determine the course that we take. As your cancer doctor, I will be your first mate. I will help you navigate these difficult waters as best as I can, though neither of us can control the storm.

The Role of Palliative Care

At some point during your treatment, your cancer doctor may say, "I would like to refer you to palliative care." If you have been referred to palliative care, please do not be scared! Palliative care is a wonderful resource that can improve your quality of life.

Palliative care is a field of medicine focused on symptom management and supportive care. You may have had prior experience with palliative care through a family member or friend with cancer. Often, the most familiar aspect of palliative care is something known as **hospice**. Hospice is an end of life program for patients with advanced cancer (you can find more information about hospice in the next section of this chapter). So you might be initially alarmed if your doctor refers you to palliative care.

However, palliative care does not always equal hospice! As mentioned, palliative care is a group of providers who focus on issues such as symptom management. Cancer is not easy to deal with. Chemotherapy is not easy to deal with. People can have symptoms from their cancer and chemotherapy such as pain, nausea, and anxiety...the list goes on and on.

As your cancer doctor, I focus on treating your cancer. However, I am also treating you as a whole person! That includes any symptoms you may be struggling with. Having palliative care as part of your treatment team means that you will have the support of doctors and nurses who specialize in improving cancer symptoms. Instead of having just one doctor helping you, now you have a whole team of providers helping you succeed.

So do not be scared! Go to your palliative care appointment, and see how your cancer team can help make your life better.

Hospice Does Not Mean Giving Up

As mentioned, hospice is an end of life service provided to patients with advanced cancer. The goal with hospice is no longer "fixing" your disease, but rather, making whatever time you have left as comfortable and as happy as possible. Typically, hospice is reserved for patients who have less than six months to live and who are no longer a candidate for chemotherapy.

There are two types of hospice services: home hospice and inpatient hospice. Home hospice is a service where you stay in your own home, and hospice employees come to your house two to three times per week to provide care. In addition, a hospice nurse will be available 24/7 by phone in case you have any urgent questions or concerns. The hospice nurse will also provide you with a medicine kit with carefully labeled medications for various symptoms.

To participate in home hospice, you must have a caregiver who can provide daily care for you. As mentioned, your hospice nurse will come to your home a couple of hours per week—however, the remainder of your care will need to be provided by family or friends. Second, you may have medical needs that exceed what can be provided in a home setting. For instance, some patients require very high levels of oxygen, certain types of suction, or types of medications that cannot be given by mouth. For these patients, inpatient hospice may be a better option. Inpatient hospice facilities are nursing facilities that have the ability to give IV medications, high flow oxygen, and suction. In order to qualify for inpatient hospice, you will need to be evaluated by a hospice provider and deemed appropriate for inpatient hospice.

Both home hospice and inpatient hospice are typically paid for through your insurance or through Medicare. Most patients and their families never have to pay out of pocket for hospice care.

Again, hospice is not about giving up. Hospice will not shorten your life. Studies have actually shown that patients with stage 4 cancer live *longer* on hospice compared to patients without hospice. This is likely because the goal with hospice is *quality of life*. When people feel better, they tend to live longer.

If you are considering hospice or interested in hearing more about hospice, talk to your oncologist. If you decide to pursue hospice, your oncologist will fully support your decision. He or she likely became a doctor with the goal of helping people. Hospice answers the question, "How can I make your life better?" when the answer is no longer "Chemotherapy."

There Is Always Hope

I am not God. At the end of the day, I do not control how long you have on this earth. When I talk about prognosis, the numbers I give you are based on clinical trials and observational studies. Some people live longer than the numbers I quote, while some people live shorter. At the end of the day, *you* are not a number. So when you look at me and ask, "Is there any hope for me?" The answer is—*yes*.

The goal with chemotherapy is to provide you with more *good quality time*. I want you to be able to spend time with your family. I want you to be able to do the things that you want to do. Gaining more time also allows time for new medical discoveries. Every day, new medications are being approved for advanced cancers. Ten years ago, immunotherapy was just emerging on the oncology scene. Now, immunotherapy is used to treat everything from skin cancer to lung cancer. Sometimes, immunotherapy can even cure cancers that were previously thought incurable.

The point is, things change with time. If I can buy you a little more time, it might be just enough time to have a miracle happen. I want you to believe, to hope that between God and science, things can change for *you*.

I know that it can be extremely difficult to find a balance between hope and realism. As mentioned before, my motto is to prepare for the worst, but hope and pray for the best. My goal is to provide you with the information you need to make plans and make the most of whatever time you have left. However, my hope is that somewhere along the journey of your cancer treatment, there may be a new mutation, a new drug, or a new chemotherapy that offers a more effective and gentler way of treating your cancer. By buying you more time with chemotherapy, I hope to provide you with the chance to benefit from these new discoveries.

Even if you are at the point in your cancer journey where you are no longer a candidate for chemotherapy; even if you are on hospice, preparing for the next and last phase of your life. Your cancer experience has made an impact on your family and friends, as well as the doctors and nurses who have cared for you. Your story may inspire another woman to get her mammogram, which in turn may end up saving her life. Your journey may inspire a neighbor to quit smoking, a nephew to get his colonoscopy—a friend to talk to her doctor about a pain that has been bothering her for the past couple of months. And though a cure has not yet been found for some cancers, every patient that we as doctors treat teaches us something new and important about this ever-changing disease. We also learn more about the resistance and strength of the human spirit, and how love, faith, and hope can bring out the best in people even during the darkest of hours. Your story inspires us to continue to strive for a cure and to hopefully, someday make cancer a thing of the past.

So yes. There is always hope.

WHAT YOU HAVE LEARNED IN THIS CHAPTER

Summary:

- Stage 4 cancer is typically treated with chemotherapy alone. The goal of chemotherapy is to increase quality as well as quantity of life.
- Typically stage 4 cancers cannot be cured.
- If you have been diagnosed with stage 4 cancer, life during treatment will different than it was prior to cancer. However, life can still be meaningful. There is always hope.
- Palliative care is a field of medicine focused on improving quality of life for patients receiving cancer treatment. If you have been struggling with symptoms from your cancer, ask your doctor about a palliative care referral.
- Hospice is an end of life service provided to patients who have advanced cancer. If your doctor has told you that you are no longer a candidate for chemotherapy, or you have decided for yourself to stop further treatment, please ask your doctor for a hospice referral.

In this chapter, I have discussed several issues that are unique to patients with stage 4 cancer. I have discussed the need to adjust your expectations for your life and for your cancer treatment. I have reminded you that though life may be difficult, there are still many things worth living for. The goal of your cancer treatment is to improve your quality of life. With that in mind, I reviewed the role of palliative care, and finally, of hospice.

Conclusion

A year later, I entered the exam room with a smile on my face. Ms. Elizabeth was back for a routine follow up exam.

"How are you doing, dear?" I asked. Ms. Elizabeth looked great. Her hair had grown back in, and she had it styled in a short, chic bob. She looked rested and relaxed.

"I'm doing fantastic," she replied. She was taking her endocrine therapy and tolerating it well. She had just had her annual mammogram, which came back normal. "I have an occasional hot flash, but I just take off whatever layers I can and keep going."

She told me that she was back at work, and she and her husband had just celebrated an anniversary by going on a cruise. Her family was doing well. "My youngest is now going to be a senior in high school," she said, laughing. "I can't believe it. And my oldest just graduated college and is about to start her Master's."

We chatted a bit more about her family and her job. After a normal examination, I refilled her endocrine medication and set her up to return to clinic in six months. "Well, I'm happy to hear everything is going well," I told her as walked towards the door. "I think that you're doing great."

She started gathering her things. "Thank you," she said with a smile. "I think I am too!"

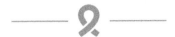

Every day, I see patients just like Ms. Elizabeth in my office. I see patients who initially walk into my office scared and overwhelmed, uncertain of what the future might bring. Together, we work to conquer those fears. Through knowledge, patience, time, and compassion, we figure out the road ahead of us. Over time, I see that fear disappear, and I see strength and confidence begin to emerge. I see patients develop a deeper understanding about their health and their life priorities. And ultimately, I see patients who are better able to navigate the future before them because they understand the journey they have already taken.

I wrote this book in the hopes that I help you on your own journey. I have tried to provide you a voice that you may not hear as often in a cancer resource book--the oncologist's perspective. My hope is that by providing you with the knowledge you needed to navigate these murky waters, you have felt empowered and equipped to handle whatever life throws at you during this difficult time.

In this book, you have learned the basics of cancer staging, treatment, and side effects, as well as insider tips and tricks to manage these side effects. I have reviewed the labs we frequently monitor, emotional, physical, and financial issues that may arise during chemotherapy, and finally, the myriad of emotionally difficult but vital concepts that accompany a stage 4 cancer diagnosis.

I hope that I have prepared you for the experience to come, and have addressed issues that can arise along the way. I hope that you feel stronger and more equipped to deal with whatever life throws at you during your treatment. Above all, no matter what your cancer type, stage, or treatment, I hope that you *thrive.*

If the information in this book helped you during your cancer journey, I am so happy to hear that! Please pass this book on to another cancer patient. There are so many individuals struggling with cancer. My hope is that someday, cancer will be a thing of the past and that no one will ever need to know anything more about chemotherapy. However, until that day, knowledge is power, and my goal is to empower every cancer patient about to embark on the difficult journey of cancer treatment.

Acknowledgements

I would like to thank my wonderful husband, Stephen, and my daughter Grace for their love, support, and encouragement. I would also like to thank my parents for their lifelong belief in me, and the many sacrifices that they made for me throughout my life. I would not be the woman I am today without your love.

I would like to thank my nurse, Bethany, for being a great friend and colleague. Our patients are incredibly lucky to have you as their nurse! I am also grateful to TidalHealth Peninsula Regional for giving me the opportunity to provide cancer care to my community and the town that I grew up in. I thank God every day for leading me back home.

Finally, thank you to every patient I have talked to, examined, and cared for over my medical career. Thank you for letting me be part of your life. This book was written for you.

About the Author

Dr. Angela DeRidder graduated from the University of Maryland, College Park with an undergraduate degree in physiology and neurobiology. She went on to complete a Master's in Public Health at the University of Maryland School of Public Health and attended medical school at the University of Maryland, Baltimore. Dr. DeRidder completed both her Internal Medicine residency and her Hematology/ Oncology fellow training at the University of Maryland Medical Center in Baltimore, MD.

Currently, she is a practicing medical oncologist caring for patients in rural Maryland. She is passionate about patient education and cancer prevention. When not working, Dr. DeRidder enjoys reading, writing, and spending time with her wonderful family.

Appendix

CONSULT APPOINTMENT AGENDA

Consult Appointment Agenda	
Type of cancer	
Stage of cancer	
Treatment options	
Treatment side effects	
Prognosis	
Things we need to do to get started with treatment	
Anticipated start date	

TRIAGE INFORMATION LIST

Triage information list	
Past medical history	
Past surgical history	
Current medications	
Allergies	
Social history	1. Marital Status - 2. Job - 3. Smoking history - 4. Alcohol consumption – 5. Street drug use –
Family history	1. Mother – 2. Father – 3. Maternal grandmother - 4. Maternal grandfather - 5. Paternal grandmother - 6. Paternal grandfather - 7. Brother – 8. Sister – 9. Son – 10. Daughter -

DR. DERIDDER'S QUESTION LIST

Dr. DeRidder's Question List
What type of cancer do I have (breast, lung, colon, bladder, etc.)?
What is my cancer stage?
What are my treatment options?
What are the treatment side effects?
What is my prognosis (both with treatment and without any treatment)?
What do we need to accomplish before we can get started with treatment?
What is my anticipated start date?

Glossary

Absolute neutrophil count (ANC) – The number of neutrophils or bacteria fighting immune cells, circulating in your blood system.

Adjuvant chemotherapy – Chemotherapy administered after surgery or radiation.

Advanced directives – A legal document that informs your loved ones and doctors what kinds of treatments you would want in the event that you are unable to communicate your wishes yourself. Also known as a "living will."

Anemia – A condition in which you do not have enough healthy red blood cells. Symptoms can include fatigue, paleness, shortness of breath, lightheadedness, dizziness, or racing heartbeat.

Ativan – An anti-anxiety medication that can also be used for nausea control. Potentially habit-forming.

Bone marrow – The spongy tissue inside your hip, spine, and thigh bones that produces your red blood cells, platelets, and immune cells.

Cancer staging – The process of determining the size and spread of your cancer.

Cannobidiol oil (CBD) - Extract of cannabis or marijuana plants. Frequently used to treat pain, nausea, insomnia, and anxiety.

Chemotherapy – Medicines administered to destroy cancer cells.

Clinical trial – A research study evaluating the effectiveness and benefit of a particular cancer treatment.

Colace - A stool softener that works by increasing the amount of water the stool absorbs in the intestines. Also known as docusate.

Compazine – A type of anti-nausea medication, also known as prochlorperazine.

Concurrent chemoradiation – Chemotherapy and radiation administered during the same time interval. Also considered **definitive therapy**.

Definitive therapy – Cancer treatment that has the potential to permanently kill cancer cells; typically involves either surgery or radiation, however, in certain types of cancers can involve chemotherapy alone.

Dexamethasone – A steroid medication that has anti-inflammatory properties; can be used to control nausea.

Dose reductions – The practice of prescribing a dose of chemotherapy *below* the dose recommended by the Federal Drug Administration (FDA for a specific cancer treatment. Typically done by your medical oncologist if you have a poor performance status or if you are experiencing excessive chemotherapy side effects.

Endocrine therapy - Medications that change hormone levels to affect cancer cells. Examples include Letrozole (Femara), anastrole (Arimidex), exemestane (Aromasin), and Tamoxifen.

Enema – A procedure in which liquid is administered into the rectum to stimulate stool evacuation.

Federal Drug Administration (FDA) – A government agency responsible for protecting the public health by ensuring the safety, efficacy, and security of human drugs, products, and medical devices.

Financial toxicity - The cumulative cost of cancer treatment, including co-pays, cost of medications, and hospital bills.

Gingivostomatitis – Viral infection of the lips and soft mucosal tissue characterized by ulcers and blisters.

Health care proxy – Individual who is authorized to make medical decisions on your behalf in the event you are unable to make medical decisions on your own. You typically identify your health care proxy in a document called "**Advanced Directives**," also known as a "living will."

Hospice - An end of life program for patients with terminal health conditions, such as cancer, who have a prognosis of less than six months.

Imodium – An anti-diarrhea medication.

Immunotherapy – A type of medicine that stimulates the immune system with the goal of having the immune system kill cancer cells.

Iron deficient – A condition in which your iron levels are below normal. Can result in **anemia**. Symptoms of iron deficiency include fatigue, weakness, paleness, dizziness, and cold hands and feet.

Lactulose – A stool softener that works by increasing the amount of water the stool absorbs in the intestines.

L-Lysine – Over the counter aminoacid supplement that can help with **gingivostomatitis**.

Lomotil – An anti-diarrhea medication.

Lymphocytes – Immune cells that help to protect you against viruses.

Magic mouthwash – A compounded prescription solution that typically contains equal parts of Benadryl, Maalox, and lidocaine (sometimes also contains Nystatin, a topical anti-fungal). Used for treatment of **mucositis**.

Magnesium citrate – A stool softener that works by increasing the amount of water the stool absorbs in the intestines.

Medical oncologist – Physician trained to administer chemotherapy for the treatment of cancer.

Metastatic – Spread of your cancer from the site of origin to another part of the body.

Miralax – A stool softener that works by increasing the amount of water the stool absorbs in the intestines.

Mucositis – Ulcers and irritation of the inside of the mouth and throat. Can be caused by chemotherapy or radiation.

National Comprehensive Cancer Network – An alliance of cancer centers dedicated to improving and facilitating quality, effective, efficient, and accessible cancer care. Develops practice guidelines for oncology providers among many other roles.

Neoadjuvant chemotherapy – Chemotherapy administered before surgery or **definitive therapy**.

Neulasta – A shot prescribed by your medical oncologist to booster up your **absolute neutrophil count**.

Neupogen – A shot prescribed by your medical oncologist to booster up your **absolute neutrophil count**. Typically 5 doses of neupogen = 1 dose of **Neulasta**.

Neutropenia, neutropenic – A condition in which your **absolute neutrophil count** is less than 1000.

Neutropenic precautions – Precautions recommended by your oncologist if your **absolute neutrophil count** is less than 1000. Geared towards minimizing your contact with bacteria and viruses.

Neutrophils – Immune cells that protect you against bacteria.

Palliative care - A field of medicine focused on symptom management and supportive care.

Performance status – A measure of your overall well-being and robustness. Generally calculated based on how able well you are able to perform your activities of daily living.

Phenergan – A type of anti-nausea medication, also known as promethazine.

Pink Ribbon Diet, the – A lifestyle regimen created by Dr. Mary Flynn, a research dietitian and assistant professor at Brown Medical School. The Pink Ribbon Diet emphasizes a plant-based, olive-oil diet that can help manage weight gain, enable better control over blood sugar and cholesterol, and improve blood pressure.

Point person – Individual designated to help disseminate information to your family and friends. Typically a verbal assignment. For some patients, this individual may also serve as a patient's emergency contact or power of attorney.

Power of attorney – Individual designated to make legal and financial decisions for you in the event that you are unable to make legal and financial decisions on your own. You identify this person in a legal document which requires witnesses and notarization.

Prior authorization – A process that some insurance companies use to encourage doctors to prescribe only certain medications, scans or procedures for a particular medical diagnosis.

Prognosis – Your chance of being alive or cancer free at a certain future time point.

Quality of life – Your overall health, comfort, and happiness.

Radiation – Energy released in the form of particles or electromagnetic waves with the goal of killing cancer cells by disrupting their DNA.

Radiation oncologist – Physician trained to administer radiation for the treatment of cancer.

Sancuso patch – A long-acting form of anti-nausea medication in the same family as Zofran. Typically worn as a patch on the skin for seven days, after which the patch is removed and replaced.

Senna – A stool softener that works by increasing contractions in the intestines to move stool out of the body. Also known as sennakot.

Spleen – An organ that sits above your stomach and under your left-sided ribs. Recycles old red blood cells, platelets, and immune cells.

Surgery – A procedure typically performed by a **surgeon** in which cancer is resected or removed from the body.

Surgical oncologist – Physician trained to performed surgical procedures to remove different types of cancer.

Survivorship – Issues related to follow-up care (such as regular health and wellness checkups), late effects of treatment, cancer recurrence, second cancers, and quality of life.

Thrombocytopenia – A condition in which you do not have enough healthy platelets. Symptoms include easy bruising or bleeding.

Thrush – A yeast infection of the mouth and throat. Can frequently occur during **chemotherapy.**

Valtrex – Prescription antiviral medication.

White blood cell count (WBC) – Your immune system. Mostly consists of neutrophils and lymphocytes.

Zofran – A type of anti-nausea medication, also known as ondansetron.

Index

A

Absolute neutrophil count (ANC)
86-90, 100-101, 231
American Cancer Society 42, 49
American Gastroenterological
Association 75
Anemia 96-98, 231
Ativan 69, 231

B

Believe 144-147
Biopsy 35, 51
Bone marrow 51, 97, 99, 101,
103

C

Calling the On-call Oncologist
what do they need to know?
84
Cancer
aggressive 12-13
Cancer staging 5-7, 36, 199,
232
stage 1 5
stage 2 5
stage 3 5
stage 4 5, 7, 196-217

finding a new normal 202-
204
Cannobidiol oil 175-177
Case manager 42, 83, 147
Chemotherapy 6-9, 15, 17, 23-
24, 108 116, 138-139, 143,
160, 163-170, 198, 199, 202,
204, 205, 207-209, 212, 214-
215
adjuvant 9-15, 231
diet 66, 72, 160-165
antioxidants 163
Pink Ribbon Diet 164-165,
167-167, 236
sugar 163
dose reductions 98, 104-108,
233
hydrate 66, 70, 168-170
labs 96-104
limbo 142
neoadjuvant 9-12, 235
oral form 148
side effects 19, 64, 90, 97,
143, 194
constipation 75-80
Constipation management
pyramid 76

Made in the USA
Monee, IL
11 May 2021